Crisis in the Community:
The African Caribbean Experience of Mental Health

By David Burke

'One million people commit suicide every year'
The World Health Organization

David Burke

Published by
Chipmunkapublishing
PO Box 6872
Brentwood
Essex CM13 1ZT
United Kingdom

http://www.chipmunkapublishing.com

Edited by Mary Dow

Crisis in the Community

"I've been 'buked and I've been scorned
I've been 'buked and I've been scorned
Children, I've been 'buked and I've been scorned
Tryin' to make this journey all alone."
'Buked and Scorned – Spiritual.

"So as a prelude Whites must be made to realise that they are only human, not superior. Same with Blacks. They must be made to realise that they are also human, not inferior."
Steven Biko.

David Burke

Crisis in the Community

For Shirley, who never stopped believing. I love you.

David Burke

Crisis in the Community

Acknowledgements

I don't recommend working full-time when taking on a book of this magnitude – not to mention embarking on a freelance journalism career, studying for a degree and raising a son who is oblivious to the sound of silence. I love you madly, Dylan, and thank you for always asking about my progress – I hope I've done you proud.

Thanks also to my wife, Shirley, for never doubting me as a writer, for her good advice, encouragement and, mostly, for her friendship. It is her beautifully evocative illustration that adorns the cover; for as well as her brilliant intellect, unfailing humanity and ability to endure my occasionally difficult personality – which alone would be sufficient as an attribute – she is an impressive artist who should really paint more than she does.

Others on the domestic front who warrant acknowledgement are Francesca (a Broadcast Journalist for the future), my sister-in-law Faye, mother-in-law Vicky, and, of course, my own parents, Gabriel and Eileen Burke.

Thanks to my friend, Jonathan Ashby, who pointed me in the direction of Chipmunka Publishing. Thanks too to Jason Pegler at Chipmunka Publishing for placing his faith in me; to Catherine Jackson, Editor of Mental Health Today, for affording me space in her magazine within which I could explore several of the issues covered here; and to Marverine Cole for giving me a platform on her BBC WM radio show to publicise *Crisis in the Community* even before a word had been written.

"And thanks to all those who kindly agreed to be interviewed: Matilda Macattram (whosewords provided the title for the book), Rameri Moukam, Maxie Hayles, Professor SumanFernando, Dr Richard Stone, Professor Kwame McKenzie, Dr Roi Kwabena (who has since sadly passed away), Devon Marston, Coral Hines, Claire Felix, Sieta Lambrias, Gilroy Brown and Bishop Joe Aldred. Finally, to Lee Walker-Wright for putting me in touch with the late Dr Kwabena."

Crisis in the Community

Prologue

I came to this project as an outsider, neither a member of the African Caribbean community or a mental health professional, but as an Irishman living in Britain acutely aware of difference, of not belonging. My community carries its own historical baggage, the relative burden of which is as oppressive as that borne by African Caribbeans. There is a sense of similar roads travelled by both communities, or as Bishop Joe Aldred, Chair of the Council of Black-Led Churches, quipped - after failing to convince me of the merits of cricket - "You and I have something in common – we were both colonised by the Brits!"

And the aftershocks of colonialism are still being felt by the progeny of the colonised, none more so than African Caribbeans. Don't subscribe to the hype generated by the New Labour Government that Britain exists as a multicultural oasis in a Europe driven by ethnic conflict. It is one of the many fallacies woven by their unremitting propagandists. They may comfort themselves with the conceit of their rectitude in reversing the bad old days of Tory rule, but the professionals, the activists, the grass roots workers, the people who live and breathe the consequences of being black in Britain every single day, know different. They know that Britain is multicultural in appearance only, that in practice if you're not White Anglo-Saxon, and especially if you're Black, you are part of a culture that is other. And on that premise you are denied, in an almost Machiavellian way, the same services, the same rights, the same respect, as the indigenous White population. This is fundamentally why African Caribbeans are over-represented in the criminal justice system and the mental health system; this is why African Caribbeans under-perform in the education system; this is why African Caribbeans are marginalised in employment; this is why African Caribbeans live in destitution on sink estate slums where drugs and guns are common currency.

Colonialism, at its most basic, was all about racism – the ascendancy of White over Black. And just as the colonised are genetically predisposed to the mental and physical struggle wrought by what Bishop Aldred calls rootlessness, the colonisers continue to abstractedly wield the whip. This is why African Caribbean men like David 'Rocky' Bennett and Michael Powell, men with mental health issues, die in the stewardship of the authorities entrusted with their care. Because they're Black.

This book is not an academic treatise on the African Caribbean experience of the mental health system. My intention is not to collate empirical evidence and statistical data, and precisely summarise in the cold-blooded language of intellect. Rather this is a manifestly subjective account of the African Caribbean experience of the mental health system by those African

Crisis in the Community

Caribbeans who are involved in and who use the system – a platform for insights far too often discounted.

David Burke 2008

David Burke

Crisis in the Community

Chapter One

"This is a crisis that's destroyed a generation of African Caribbeans. Look at our community. Look at the children on the streets. Look at what's happening. Of all immigrant groups, look at the state we're in. Mental health services have done incredible amounts of damage to Black people in Britain today."

These indignant words are spoken by Matilda Macattram of Black Mental Health UK, an organisation dedicated to raising awareness of what is broadly accepted as the disproportionate treatment of Britain's African Caribbean community within the mental health system.

In January 2005, the Department of Health published a five-year action plan, *Delivering Race Equality in Mental Health Care*, the aim of which was to achieve equality and tackle discrimination where it exists in mental health services in England. The five-year action plan set out the Government's response to the recommendations made by the independent inquiry into the death of David 'Rocky' Bennett, a 38-year-old African Caribbean inpatient in a medium secure psychiatric unit in Norwich. It emphasised the need for more appropriate and responsive services, a programme for engaging the community and better information from improved monitoring of ethnicity. The intention was to help providers of mental health services to ensure they were meeting the standards defined in *National Standards, Local Action*. Two core standards were particularly relevant: that healthcare organisations must challenge discrimination, promote equality and respect human rights and that organisations must enable all members of the population to access services equally. One of the key components of the plan was the inception of a national yearly census of inpatients in mental health hospitals and facilities in England and Wales. The objectives of *Count Me In: The National Mental Health and Ethnicity Census* were to obtain reliable information about the number of inpatients using mental health services and to encourage all providers of mental health services to have accurate, comprehensive and sustainable procedures for collecting, recording and monitoring ethnicity that would permit them to collect data of a high quality on the ethnicity of patients. A third objective was to investigate the extent to which providers of mental health care have implemented culturally sensitive, appropriate and responsive services with effective care planning and local evaluation, influenced by information on the ethnicity of patients.

As Professor Sir Ian Kennedy and Professor Lord Kamlesh Patel wrote in the foreword to the initial report, "It is wrong and intolerable if someone is categorised as mentally ill and hospitalised solely on the basis of colour or ethnic origin. It is equally wrong and intolerable if someone who is mentally ill and would benefit from care in hospital did not

Crisis in the Community

have that benefit because those charged with such decisions are anxious that they may be accused of racial prejudice. Patients should receive care appropriate to their needs, reducing the need for hospitalisation and detention where appropriate."

The census, conducted jointly by the Healthcare Commission, the Mental Health Act Commission and the National Institute for Mental Health (England), collected details of ethnicity, language and religion, as well as a range of information about how each inpatient came to be in hospital and details of their care. The first annual results revealed an alarming pattern of disparity in how the system deals with African Caribbeans. In short, the findings illustrated that African Caribbeans were three times more likely than the average to be admitted to a psychiatric hospital, 44% more likely to be detained under the Mental Health Act, twice as likely to be referred through the courts, 50% more likely to be placed in seclusion once in hospital and 29% more likely to experience incidents involving physical restraint. Furthermore, they were 70% less likely to be referred by a GP for counselling and other non-institutional rehabilitation treatments.

The figures made for stark reading. Evidently the mental health system was, as had been suggested by activists within the African Caribbean community for at least three decades, failing to deliver equitable care to said community.

This was acknowledged by Professor Christopher Heginbotham, Chief Executive of the Mental Health Act Commission, who asserted that the results, "Challenge many assumptions about the nature of care". He continued, "Black and mixed heritage groups expressed views and perceptions that suggest services are failing seriously to provide relevant, supportive, respectful care and that service users are wary of professional attitudes. These matters cannot be left to resolve themselves; all commissioners and providers of mental health services must take heed, and the actions listed in *Delivering Race Equality* should be given urgent attention."

Lee Jasper, Chair of the African Caribbean Mental Health Commission, was less euphemistic; for him, the conclusions depicted a mental health service that was comparable to one, "In an institutionally racist state". He added, "Those facts are horrendous. What's missing from the Government is any acceptance that institutionalised racism is driving these figures. Would you send your mother, if she were Black, to a mental health institution? Not on these figures. I'd take them to a church or find some other means. The figures are so bad they are reflective of a mental health system almost in an apartheid state. I'd like to compare these figures with the mental health system in South Africa during apartheid."

Crisis in the Community

The 2006 census results, published in the second year of the DRE programme, showed no discernible change, with African Caribbean patients again disproportionately detained compared to other groups, placed in seclusion more, and subjected to greater control and restraint. Reverend Pedro Emmanuel, Chair of the African Caribbean Evangelical Alliance, accused the Government of "paying lip service" to the very real concerns of the African Caribbean lobby in relation to mental health. "This is not acceptable in 21st Century Britain," he said. "We all have a stake and we cannot be treated as second-rate citizens because of our colour. The death of David Bennett should have marked a watershed, but sadly it is to the contrary."

Why is the mental health system failing its African Caribbean service users? And why are these same service users "wary of professional attitudes"? Is it simply cultural insensitivity, or something altogether more insidious? Could there really be a covert policy of apartheid at work here, as intimated by Jasper?

The panel which oversaw the *Independent Inquiry into the Death of David Bennett* certainly thought race was the main factor. Its findings determined that the mental health system was institutionally racist. The term was first coined by American civil rights activist Stokely Carmichael in 1967, who explained, "If a church is bombed and five Black children die, that's individual racism. But when

5,000 Black babies die each year from lack of food, decent shelter and no medical care, that's institutional racism."

It was applied in a British context to the Metropolitan Police by Sir William Macpherson, who oversaw the inquiry into the death of Stephen Lawrence, a young Black man attacked and murdered by a gang of White males at a bus stop in South London in 1993. Essentially he identified as "the collective failure of an organisation to provide an appropriate and professional service to people because of their colour, culture or ethnic origin. It can be seen as detected in processes, attitudes and behaviour which amount to discrimination through unwitting prejudice, ignorance, thoughtlessness and racist stereotyping, which disadvantage minority ethnic people".

But the Government didn't accept the Bennett inquiry's recommendation - one of 17 contained in the inquiry report – much to the disappointment of Dr Richard Stone, a member of the inquiry panel. "It was heartbreaking to have our two key recommendations rejected by the Secretary of State and the Health Minister," he recalls now. "These were the acceptance of institutional racism and a limit on restraint of a patient of three minutes. A year later (following publication of the report), the Department of Health proposed restraint only for as long as absolutely necessary. Yet that is what five nurses who killed 'Rocky' Bennett had been taught in their restraint training."

Crisis in the Community

Indeed John Reid, Health Secretary at the time of publication of the inquiry report, was adamant the Government wouldn't be persuaded by the institutional racism recommendation. Lord Patel, former National Director of *Delivering Race Equality*, said Reid felt, "It let people off the hook. He was arguing that once you say it is institutional racism, people will say, 'It's nothing to do with me', and you can't do anything about it".

Even as New Labour's propensity for occasionally perplexing spin goes, Reid's reasoning stretches every sinew of credibility. Accepting a recommendation by an esteemed panel of mental health professionals that racism is endemic within the system would be tantamount to absolving the perpetrators of any wrongdoing, and furthermore would inhibit progress. Small wonder that with such unique political acumen, Reid failed to ever find his ministerial niche. In one way though perhaps Reid was right, however unintentionally. Racism is, after all, not merely confined to institutions; it is the scourge of society. Bishop Joe Aldred, Chair of the Council of Black-Led Churches, puts it more succinctly. "I think the issue of institutional racism is a factor in all services. It's a pity that we keep on picking off service by service. It would be nice if we could just recognise that Europeans have a view of Black people, and Black people have an experience of living amongst Europeans, the result of which is what is called institutional racism. "Services are developed and administered in a way that is not sympathetic towards Black people; and Black people's experience of trying to access those services is one that is always fraught with difficulty. So in that regard mental health is no different to education or to other aspects of health – or to trying to get a bus! I actually don't make a big issue of it other than it is there. It is a symptom of an historical legacy, partly of slavery, partly of the slave trade, partly of Black and White encounters in Africa and what ensued in the Caribbean. It is there and it plays out within these institutions."

Crisis in the Community

Chapter Two

Health is defined by the World Health Organisation as "a state of complete physical, mental and social wellbeing, and not merely the absence of disease or infirmity". The pre-requisites for health include peace, shelter, education, food, income, a stable economy, sustainable resources, social justice and equal opportunity for all. According to Mind, the National Association for Mental Health, the African Caribbean community is disproportionately disadvantaged in most, if not all, of the above.

The National Institute for Mental Health (NIMHE) offers the explanation that inequalities have existed within the NHS since its foundation in 1948 because the British welfare state has ignored issues of discrimination. The assumption was that standard services would be provided for those in need, yet evidence in two 1998 reports uncover clear inequalities in the provision of healthcare, particularly to women, old people, the working class and Black and Minority Ethnic groups. NIMHE claims that this is the case because certain groups do not start from a level playing field. Society categorises people by a range of social divisions, including male, female, skin colour, age, sexual orientation or disability; and in forming a perception of them, they are pigeonholed by society, which adapts a behaviour and attitude to them in terms of how they are classified.

David Burke

People of African origin have lived in Britain for at least two millennia, arriving many hundreds of years before the forced migrations sparked by the slave trade and British colonisation. In Roman times, for example, Black troops were sent to the remote province of Britannia, some of them remaining behind when the Roman legions quit Britain. Later, in the Middle Ages, the Moors – Muslims who conquered Spain in the 8th Century – came; the word 'Moors' was also used to denote natives of Morocco or Mauritania in North Africa and in Britain, often referred to anyone of Black origin.

Of course, the number of Africans and those of African descent increased markedly with the advent of the slave trade, British involvement in which began in the 16th Century. Estate owners from the West Indies brought their household slaves to Britain to work as servants. In other instances, slaves were traded on these shores, often through newspaper advertisements. In 1756, for example, the *Liverpool Advertiser* carried a request for a, "Black boy of deep Black complexion... not above fifteen nor under twelve years of age".

Not all Black people who lived in Britain during this period were enslaved. Africans were recruited as sailors on the numerous slaving voyages of British traders, and it is likely that some of these sailors were free men. And some Africans were, in fact,

Crisis in the Community

merchants here on business, while many were the children of wealthy African rulers or European planters who sought education in Europe. One of these was Francis Williams, a Jamaican of African descent who studied at Cambridge University in the early 1700s and who, on his return to the West Indies, operated a school in Spanish Town, Jamaica.

Although specific numbers are difficult to ascertain – the first national census wasn't conducted until 1801 and even that was limited in scope – in 1764, *Gentleman's Magazine* estimated that 20,000 Black people lived in London alone. In 1772, Lord Mansfield, whose judgement in the Somerset case held that slavery was unlawful in England (though not elsewhere in the British Empire) and was heralded as a significant milestone in the campaign to abolish slavery, put the number in the country as a whole at 15,000.

Images of Black people were common in British art and culture from the first days of the slave trade. In the 16th Century, masks of Black faces were worn in court society at fashionable functions and pageants and members of the aristocracy painted themselves Black. The Black Moor featured in plays by Shakespeare, while London street names included Black Boy Court and Blackmoor's Alley.

By the 18th Century, images of Black people represented prosperity and high fashion; trade cards featuring Africans promoted commodities such as tobacco, spices, tea and coffee. Black children were bought and pampered like pets by wealthy White families, and Black servants and soldiers became symbols of social standing. Yet there was a trophy element to all of this, with Britain's White populace using Blackness as a means of displaying ostentation and power, based on ideas of racial superiority. Such ideas were expressed more overtly during the reign of Elizabeth I, with some writers depicting Blackness as Satanic and sinful, and Whiteness as pure and virginal, attributes ostensibly possessed by the monarch herself. A more extreme manifestation of racism emerged; cartoonist Robert Cruikshank, among others, was responsible for disseminating distorted and grotesque images of Black people. Their physical characteristics and skin colour in these cartoons were symptomatic of their supposed mental inferiority and laziness. Writers such as Edward Long denied the humanity of Black people; hundreds of books and tracts defined Black people in absurd ways, while proclaiming the civilised nature and intellectual supremacy of Whites, which thus gave them the right to rule.

Ignatius Sancho, a distinguished man of letters whom educated White society found considerably more palatable than most Black people, acknowledged, in 1780, "The national antipathy and prejudice towards the British people's woolly-headed brethren". He complained that, to Whites,

Crisis in the Community

Blacks were, "Either foolish or mulish, all without a single exception".

In the late 19th Century, the concept of scientific racism, which drew on physical anthropology, anthropometry, craniometry, phrenology and other now discredited disciplines to justify the slave trade, purported to show evolutionary discrepancies between races or ethnic groups. Or, put simply, it alleged that Blacks were less evolved than Whites.

Renowned consultant psychiatrist Professor Suman Fernando suggests that the disciplines of psychiatry, psychology and sociology emerged when colonisation and slavery were at their peak. The view that Black people were born with inferior brains and had limited capacity for growth and that their personalities tended to be abnormal due to genetic and environmental factors was deemed normal. Long-standing prejudice based on concepts of race – principally skin colour race – became integrated as racism into Euro-American culture, including the culture of psychiatry and psychology, he contends. Observations by psychiatrists in the United States during slavery were unambiguous in maintaining that psychiatry helped to reinforce racism and justify the subjugation of Black people. Slaves who fled captivity were diagnosed as having draptomania, a disease invented by Dr Samuel Cartwright, a specialist at the University of Louisiana. The treatment meted out to them was their return to captivity and bondage.

The enduring effects of slavery must never be underestimated. The enforced displacement of Black people from Africa and their brutal relocation to the so-called New World, their relegation to subservient status, continues to haunt their descendants, just as it gives residual weight to those Whites who perpetuate the pre-eminence of their race.

Bishop Aldred believes the European notion of Black people, "Is so terribly distorted by the experience of chattel slavery especially". He explains, "The experience on both sides: the experience of the slave traders and the plantation owners, and the information that was fed into mainstream British society about the nature of Black people; and the experience of Black people who have suffered at the hands of Whites. We have a legacy of White perception of Black, Black perception of White, and Black perception of Black which need to be addressed. We have to find a way of joining up how we address this largely educational process of changing perceptions across all these zones. Otherwise, if we try it within particular disciplines, you have limited success. We have to look across the macro existence we all share and actually try to see what we can do in a joined up way to change perceptions. At the same time, of course, we have to look at what is happening and take steps within mental health. One of the ways of doing this is to ensure that Black people are involved in the development of services and in the delivery of services. Even where you don't have Black professionals, seek Black advice. "The challenge we have is that of inclusiveness of the approach to the development and delivery of services. We have to work hard at it. There is a role for Black people. It's not just about White people. Black people need to go on the offensive and develop a more militant approach towards the services we receive across the board. We very often just take what we get. We have historically just voted Labour. Why? Labour should earn the vote of a Black person the same as anyone else. We need to become more sophisticated in how we vote; far more sophisticated in the way we deal with mental health trusts and with clinicians. You should be offered choice in what service you get, how you get it, where you get it. We need to be aware of this. People aren't going to give you power. We have to empower ourselves and empower each other. You may be suffering from mental illness, but you can still walk about with the sense that you're a fully fledged human being. And if you don't feel you're being treated with the appropriate dignity, then complain. This country is racist, but it's more classist. So a Black person, who is articulate and knows their way around the services, will get the best services."

*

David Burke

The post-war economic migrants who travelled to Britain from the West Indies in 1948 – known as the Windrush generation after the SS Empire Windrush which brought 500 of them here – encountered a sometimes hostile environment. National Archive files chronicle the true extent of loathing and discrimination they faced, with virulently racist attitudes notably rampant in the police force. Officers in almost twenty London boroughs submitted reports which described the immigrants as, "Unemployable owing to their uncouth behaviour and arrogant, wholly uncivilised manner". Other references described them as "dirty", "lazy", and as, "Cunning unprincipled crooks living on women and their wits".

Mixed race relationships were adjudged dangerous, with one policeman, writing in 1952, complaining, "Unfortunately, as the law stands at present, it is difficult to obtain sufficient evidence to bring these loathsome creatures before the courts." Another entry expressed concern that the country was beset by benefit fraudsters. "There is little doubt that the men, having found the land flowing with milk and honey, are urging their families and kindred to join them and partake of the benefits so loosely obtainable here," one officer stated. "What this will mean in the future I dread to think, if they breed at the same prolific rate as in their own countries." The contention among many immigrants that they were victims of racial discrimination was met with short shrift. An officer at Albany Street station in inner London

Crisis in the Community

had the impression, "That these men are obsessed with a colour bar complex, and when they are spoken to on any matter they are very difficult to deal with, preferring to make allegations of colour prejudice, which they do loudly and persistently". A chief inspector in Brixton was prepared to tacitly accept, "A certain amount of prejudice on the part of a small section of the White population", adding that, "Some employers of labour are reluctant to engage coloured personnel".

The often antagonistic reception compounded African Caribbeans' sense of rootlessess, says Bishop Aldred. And it is this same rootlessness which he diagnoses as a contributory symptom to the myriad problems African Caribbeans have been experiencing in Britain ever since. "The African Caribbean population of this country came here from the Caribbean, having been transplanted there forcibly in the first place from Africa. You've got this group of people in the Caribbean who are still, I think, trying to sort out their identity: 'Who on earth are we?' Then, of course, you bring that to England. Look at the kind of people who came here in the 1960s – they were poor people, ill-equipped to deal with the sophisticated society into which they were now coming. In the main you didn't get bright people leaving the Caribbean to come here. The majority of people who came were, like my parents, poor, many of them semi-illiterate; we came here from the bottom end of the socio-economic scale in the

Caribbean. It was economic migration that brought here. You have a whole swathe of people who don't necessarily have all the social skills to handle the racism they're faced with full frontal here. Their experience of White people back in the Caribbean was generally seeing them as superior rather than their equal. They had children. I think if you look at that historical journey from Africa, from Asia, from the Caribbean, then you get a group of largely poor people coming here immediately faced with cold climate and cold reception, Enoch Powell talking about 'rivers of blood' - what people have met is a great trauma. So it isn't that surprising to me that many of us just can't quite get to grips with it. We haven't quite sorted out our own identity, our own nationality, our own history. A lot of people simply can't cope. It's a melting pop of instability. You go for a job, you can't get the job; or you get the job, and you have to do the most menial thing within that job. I think a lot of people are just suffering from rootlessness. Our community largely, still, is a rootless community. People came here through economic aspiration. If you talk to those people they will tell you that they came for five years, to earn enough money to go back. They got stuck here and couldn't send enough money back to look after the family, and build a nest egg. That sense of rootlessness is only just now evolving into some clearer sense of, 'Well, I'm not going to go home'."

Crisis in the Community

And so those who left the Caribbean to seek their fortune in Britain, never intending to stay longer than was necessary, had no choice but to become assimilated into a society that regarded them with at best suspicion and at worst resentment. As their family structures then took shape, the problem of identity was accentuated for subsequent generations, born in Britain to Caribbean natives whose ancestral roots were torn from Africa. Bishop Aldred illustrates this predicament by citing his own children's relationship with Jamaica, the place of his birth.

"My children go to Jamaica; they don't feel at home there. They want to jump on a plane and go back to Britain. Then they come back to Birmingham and they're called a Blackie or asked, 'When are you going to go home?' People like me and my children, especially them, are best positioned to adopt a hybrid identity of Caribbean-British, a bit like African American. The problem with that is many people from the Caribbean see Africa as home, and if there's going to be a hybrid then Africa has to be in it. In that regard it would be African-British or African-English. The truth is that most Caribbean people only think about Africa in a very idealised sense. When they meet real Africans the relationship ain't exactly cosy for the most part. There is a flaw in this line then. If you go for this African-British or African-English, where's your Caribbean identity? Among a lot of my friends, the argument we're having about it is that even if they buy into the idea of being British and something else, they can't bring themselves in the first place to have the Caribbean displace Africa. You can't have African Caribbean-British. But worse than that is that most of us can't bring ourselves to calling ourselves British. And worse still we definitely can't call ourselves English. I think the Caribbean just messed us all up. You don't have anything pure in the Caribbean. We all have some crossover of some other ethnic group in our lineage. So I'm not surprised that whenever there is a breakdown and we have a massive breakdown within the African Caribbean community that a lot of us are going to struggle mentally, psychologically."

But shouldn't things be getting better for African Caribbeans given their status as one of the longer established ethnic groupings in a once monocultural society? "There are two prongs to this," says Bishop Aldred.
"There is, on the one hand, a section of the African Caribbean community which is doing very well thank you. We no longer have that monolithic poor group. What we have is a much more mixed society of African Caribbean people. Many of the children of those first migrants have gone on to university. You have an emerging middle class who, even when their family units don't function well, still have the social skills to survive and to do well in many cases. But you still have that other strain who, for myriad reasons, still have not socialised, come to terms with who they are. And if they don't have a job or a family network, they are going to find that, as soon as the pressure is

Crisis in the Community

on, they have mental problems. The system eventually gets a hold of you, and the experience we then have within that system is that most of the practitioners are White; they now come with their Eurocentric model. Most African Caribbeans have an exuberant way of behaving, and of course that's exacerbated when you have some other difficulty you're dealing with; and the reception you can get is to be viewed as someone who is far more problematic than if you were White. So even though there is an emerging African Caribbean class, we have not yet tipped the balance yet in making this other group a minority, and therefore easier to cope with." Bishop Aldred concedes there is onus on Black church leaders to be proactive in redressing this balance. "We see it as our responsibility to take issue with issues of health, for example. A number of us now work with politicians and other people within the power structure. We do think that we can do that because we are regarded within the community as honest brokers. I hope we recapture that sense of Caribbean-ness. There is something going on there which is not always evident on the surface, an attachment with back home and also here. I think there are dots that need to be joined up better than they are. The challenge is how do we do that without becoming isolationist? How do we become a greater one, a greater whole as Caribbean people without separating ourselves even further from mainstream society and making our problems even worse?"

David Burke

African Caribbeans in Britain, as several interviewees for this book told me, have been researched to death. There are whole paper mountains of statistics that demonstrate how badly they fare within the socio-economic and political framework that constitutes the World Health Organisation's criteria for positive health. Many studies conducted in the 1970s, 1980s and 1990s consistently highlighted African Caribbeans' experience of racism. Even now it is calculated that up to 20,000 African Caribbeans are physically assaulted every year. Research carried out by Gus John Associates between 2000 and 2001 pointed to inordinate treatment of African Caribbeans in the criminal justice system. They were more likely to be acquitted than White defendants, which implied they were being unnecessarily charged. The Crown Prosecution Service was more likely to object to bail for male and female African Caribbeans compared to Whites, largely on the basis that African Caribbeans were likely "to obstruct justice".

In cases which could be tried by magistrates or juries, African Caribbeans were more likely to opt for jury trial. More cases against African Caribbean defendants were discontinued on review, which again suggested that they were being charged inappropriately by police. African Caribbeans were also disproportionately affected by the stop-and-search policy. A 2004 report by the Metropolitan Police Authority found that the practice was "influenced by racial bias", indicating

Crisis in the Community

that Black people were four times more likely to be stopped than White people.

In education, the 2007 Wanless Report, compiled by the Department of Education and Skills, found that Black pupils were routinely punished more harshly, praised less and told off more often than other pupils. Staff in many schools were unwittingly racist, with Black youngsters three times more likely than White pupils to be expelled permanently. Every year 1,000 Black pupils were permanently excluded and nearly 30,000 suspended. "Exclusions are to education what stop-and-search is to criminal justice," the report concluded, going on to describe it as an "iconic issue" for those of African Caribbean heritage. The response to race equality legislation by many schools, local authorities and even part of the department itself, ranged from "grudging minimum compliance to open hostility". Other significant findings revealed that Black pupils were 1.5 times more likely than White pupils to be classified with behaviour-related special needs; that Black pupils out-performed White pupils in school entry tests, yet when these were changed to teacher observations the pattern was reversed; and that Black pupils were disproportionately placed in bottom sets because of their behaviour rather than their ability.

Spot the difference between the Wanless findings and those of the Rampton Report published by the Department of Education and Science 22 years earlier, which stated that the curriculum failed Black boys in particular, that teachers had low expectations of Black children, and that Black boys were over-represented in terms of expulsions. In employment, African Caribbeans were twice as likely to be jobless as Whites, according to a 2004 TUC report. Many of those actually in work continued to be employed in low paid and insecure jobs, earning lower wages compared to the national average, while those with either good or excellent qualifications still had greater difficulty than White counterparts with similar qualifications in gaining the most sought after positions. Trade unionists blamed exclusion from the jobs market for the ghettoisation of Black youth. TUC Race Equality Officer Roger McKenzie said, "It's outrageous that employers are allowed to discriminate against ethnic minorities like this. It is this sort of discrimination that ensures ethnic minorities are ghettoised and kept in poorly paid menial labour."

A 2003 Cabinet Office study, *Ethnic Minorities and the Labour Market,* added up the total financial cost of being Black in Britain – over £120,000. On average, Black men earn £50 less per week than White men; over a lifetime – 18 to 65 - this equates to £122,000.

The *2005 Black Manifesto*, a radical policy document compiled by a coalition of Black-led organisations outlining the political, social and economic demands of Britain's Black communities from a domestic and international perspective,

Crisis in the Community

found that one third of African Caribbeans' households lived in the most deprived wards in England. The document stated, "Historically, direct and indirect discrimination has been rife in the allocation of housing. Racial disadvantage has developed through a cycle of deprivation and lack of investment. Black people disproportionately live in poor, run-down property, in overcrowded conditions and on many of the worst local authority estates. Regeneration of these areas has been aimed at buildings and not always at people. Black people often end up excluded and marginalised." In addition, a disproportionate number of Black households figured in the homelessness registers of local authorities. More recently, the rise in house prices meant that many people from Black communities couldn't get their foot on the housing ladder. Hardly a level playing surface at all then. And hardly surprising, given the enormity of the disadvantage with which African Caribbeans are confronted on a daily basis, that so many of them suffer poor mental health.

Rameri Moukam is Clinical Director of Pattigift, the African-centred psychiatric hospital for African Caribbeans in Birmingham. Registered by the Health Commission in 2005, it was the first institution of its kind anywhere in Britain. She, like Bishop Aldred, sees identity, or the absence of, as the source of the African Caribbean demographic's trauma.

"It's something about the assimilation, something about what happened between the two communities that is actually quite destructive for us, psychologically. And that was because we don't have a sense of who we are," she says. "And then being completely overwhelmed by another identity, and then having the glass ceiling placed on top of that. The reality is you're told one thing and what you're experiencing and what you're feeling is completely different. And then you're told what you feel and experience isn't right. Of course you're going to be fucking mad! You've got to be mad, you have. We, as Black people, are depressed. We live in a state of depression. And on top of that we are more prone to becoming psychotic."

The whole foundation on which British society is grounded, Moukam alleges, is that Black people are inferior. "Most White people feel they're innately superior to Black people. If you're Black, no matter what it is you do, you're just a Black person, and you're nothing."

Crisis in the Community

Chapter Three

The struggle for equality within mental health services may have gathered pace since the turn of the century, particularly since the inquiry into the tragic death of David Bennett, but it began in the seventies. Among those involved in the early days was Rameri Moukam. She trained as a psychiatric nurse between 1975 and 1978, around which time, "The issue of Black mental health didn't enter the picture at all". It was an Irish colleague who brought to her attention the over-representation of Black patients on the psychiatric ward at St Giles' Hospital in London. Moukam remembers, "What was striking was the fact that, even though I was a nurse at that hospital, it hadn't registered with me. We, as Black people, are assimilated – African Caribbeans in particular. We don't have a language to protect ourselves from a European influence. Plus, we were in an environment – not just here, but in the Caribbean – where the European was the epitome of everything you wanted to be. When you become a professional you learn a set of criteria. It's the European criteria. You leave your Blackness at the door. Lennox Thomas talks about it as "the proxy self". When they developed an intercultural psychotherapy model, he began to think that we had a kind of split – the Black person splits themselves and they have a part that they take to the world, and a part that they have at home. There's the self they have at home and there is the proxy self they have outside. It was my proxy self that was the nurse. So you don't take your Blackness into consideration. It's like you become colourless. People talk about providing a colour blind approach. That's what we were doing – we were developing a colour blind approach. All you're doing is looking at diagnoses and you treat everybody the same, regardless of colour. Back in the seventies and early eighties, that's what you did. So the whole idea of culture and difference didn't even start to come to the fore." Moukam and a small group of people set up a charity, a sort of befriending service, and trained volunteers to go into psychiatric hospitals to support Black patients. "We'd do the basics, the stuff that people might talk about in terms of cultural awareness. You'd comb their hair, make sure they had the right kinds of combs, and make sure they had some food. It was that basic. We devised the training package for volunteers, taught them a little bit about mental health, a little bit about the drugs the clients were taking, how the hospital worked and so forth. It was nothing to do with medical input at all. The only input we gave was in terms of giving them an understanding of what a delusion was, what a hallucination was. They'd know how to look after themselves; they'd know not to push there and to push there. It was literally about befriending. The more the befrienders went on ward rounds, the more they would challenge the kind of treatment being given to Black patients. "Does this person need to be on this medication? They don't like it". They started to challenge the medical staff. It wasn't part of their brief at the time, it just happened. They were advocating on the client's behalf."

It became apparent to Moukam and her collective that all was not well in the state of Black mental health. They secured funding from the Greater London Council to investigate further, and enlisted the services of consultant psychiatrist Sashi Sashidharan and mental health activist Errol Francis. "At the time Sasha and Errol were focusing on misdiagnosis. In fact, there were a lot of cultural issues that were creating the problem for Black people in mental health and these cultural issues were being misinterpreted as symptoms. Language is part of that. For example, Jamaican Patois. There are expressions in Jamaican Patois which can be misinterpreted. Also, Black people, when they start to get ill, there's this God stuff that goes on. That can also be misinterpreted. They started to talk about getting psychiatrists trained and bringing attention to the fact that maybe there's something going on here. I don't truly believe the misdiagnosis bit. I always believed there was more to it than that. I thought there was something going on with us, that there was something about this community that was actually quite disturbing for us, for our psyche. So Black mental health got put on the map. People began to think about Black mental health, that there was something going on. We began to look at all that. There was lots of research around what was happening, what our experience was. They found things like we were being massively over-medicated - and still are – and that we were catching the hard end of the psychiatric experience all the time. We wanted to prove that all of this was actually a reality that we weren't just making it up."

Moukam eschewed the misdiagnosis theory put forward by Sashidharan and Francis; she immersed herself in psychotherapeutic work in trying to understand what was "underneath it all". She looked at things from a more socio-political as well as a medical perspective. "I thought about what was going on because of the community that meant we were suffering as we were in this country while we were going mad. Because we were going mad, there's no two ways about it. We are going mad. Still. We're going mad. And we're going mad here more so than we are anywhere else. Black people were better mentally under apartheid than they have been here." But surely Moukam must have subscribed to the misdiagnosis theory at some stage as being a contributory factor to the disproportionate treatment of African Caribbeans within the mental health system? "Yes, but that's not what gets us into psychiatric hospitals. It's more historical. Once we get in there, the hospitals have their inner culture. There's institutional racism within the psychiatric hospitals, and there's racism outside in the community. So I wasn't going where everybody else was going with the misdiagnosis thing. I understood that, but I'm not

Crisis in the Community

interested in what White people are doing - I'm more interested in what we are doing. We began to look at that whole internalised racism thing and we then begin to do it to ourselves. Internalised racism became my thing. We no longer need White people to oppress us, we do it ourselves. We don't trust ourselves, we don't trust each other. It's like a union – divide and rule. We are so disintegrated as a community and we have nothing to ground ourselves on because we were so taken away from our African roots that we're wandering around in the middle of nowhere. It just takes a couple of knocks and we're completely off the rails."

It is Bishop Joe Aldred's hypothesis of rootlessness again, a legacy of slavery, what American academic Dr Joy DeGruy Leary calls post-traumatic slave syndrome. The philosophy of Moukam's Pattigift recognises the psychological effects of Black people's history of enslavement, colonisation and institutional racism. Members are encouraged to explore all aspects of themselves in an attempt to comprehend how the internal, external, spiritual and mundane all play a part in their mental distress. "For us, it's about a complete lack of identity. And then being completely overwhelmed by another identity and having the glass ceiling on top of that. The reality is you're told one thing and what you're experiencing and what you're feeling is completely different. And then you're told that what you feel and experience isn't right. Of course you're going to be fucking mad. You've got to be mad. You have! Black people's norm is a psychotic scale. We are depressed. We live in a state of depression. And on top of that, we become psychotic. We are more prone to being psychotic." Pattigift's aspiration is to help the African Caribbean community to re-educate themselves about their identity. "In a nutshell, who the hell are we? Who told us we were that? And do we accept it? And if we don't, how then do we identify ourselves? And the way to identify ourselves is not about how much bling we have. It's about, what does this all mean? African culture says that our lives are about what we do and how that then influences the community – I am, therefore we are. That's completely different to the Eurocentric model – I think, therefore I am. That's all about the individual; we're all about the collective. We have to get back to that notion of the collective. We've taken on the Eurocentric model; we have to get back to the African model. People need to make a decision to understand why they do what they're doing, and why it is they're playing into other people's hands. All White people have to do is to change the criteria and we're fucked. So if we, as Black people, create our own criteria, we're not fucked. We have to decide how we're going to function." It's an impressive ideal – the empowerment of African Caribbeans with a sense of who they are, where they come from, what they can be. "It's about moving more and more into the community. We almost need to catch people street by street. If we can engage youth workers into thinking from this perspective, they can help the youth to see from this perspective, we will revitalise the community to understand their position, who they are and empower them to work out exactly who and what they are. There's a lot of deconstruction to reconstruct. Then we need to empower Black nurses to use their Black selves within those institutions. Once we start doing that it completely changes how people experience racism. That means we actually start to provide some real care, because all we're doing now is housing them, restraining them and medicating them. We need to get the care element back into it. You need to teach them how to use talking therapies, how to engage with people in a meaningful way."

Moukam contests that the colour blind approach, when it comes to mental health services, doesn't work; it means not dealing with the service user as an individual, it means not seeing their experience as different and so consequently treating that experience in the same way as those of other service users. It is Moukam claims, innately racist. "Of course, you can apply the same claim to other ethnic minorities - all of us. The thing that shocks people is that the mental health system doesn't do anyone any good. It's crap at the moment. But it's even more crap for Black people. It's not that they're giving White people this fantastic service and they're giving Black people a terrible one; the whole thing's crap."

Putting it bluntly, Moukam believes it's incumbent on Black people "to really deal with our shit" – and this means self-imposed segregation from White society. "We don't deal with our shit because we're having to worry about pissing off the White folk. And God we piss off the white folk – even if we ignore them we piss them off! We need time to really look at ourselves and to figure out what the hell's really going on. It's not about separating; it's about separating for a while in order to understand ourselves. It's seriously about empowering the Black community. Psychotherapy for Black people is a political act, it's pure militancy. Surviving for Black people is a political act. The thing about psychotherapy is to know thyself. If you know thyself, then you are empowered to do what it is you need to do."

In the meantime, African Caribbean service users continue to suffer within mental health services, although Moukam feels there is a sea change happening. "We're beginning to have an impact in that our existence is making them have to look seriously at what it is they're doing. And also, we now have access directly into the wards. This is the biggest time for us. If we don't get this right now in this climate, it's never happening again."

Crisis in the Community

Chapter Four

In 2002, the Sainsbury Centre for Mental Health, a registered charity working to improve the quality of life for people with mental health problems, published a report which characterised the relationship between the Black community and the mental health system as one predicated on fear. *Breaking the Circles of Fear* outlined that Black people had an overwhelmingly negative experience of mental health services, yet were not accessing the primary care, mental health promotion and specialist community services which were designed to help service users.

Dr Shirley Tate, Chair of the *Breaking the Circles of Fear* steering group, wrote at the time, "Black people mistrust and often fear services where there are truly circles of fear. Black people mistrust and often fear services and staff are often wary of the Black community, fearing criticism and not knowing how to respond and fearful of young Black men. The cycle is fuelled by prejudice, misunderstanding, misconceptions and sometimes racism."

The report indicated that the need for changes to the mental health care and treatment of Black people was, "Widely recognised and long overdue". There was, "Compelling research and statistic evidence," showing the community's over-representation within the system and comparably poorer outcomes than their White counterparts.

David Burke

Contributory factors to the way in which mental health services assessed and responded to the needs of Black and African Caribbean communities were informed by "Stereotypical views of Black people, racism, cultural ignorance, and the stigma and anxiety often associated with mental illness". When prejudice and the fear of violence influenced risk assessments and decisions on treatment, responses were likely to be dominated by a heavy reliance on medication and restriction. Service users became reluctant to ask for help or to comply with treatment, thus increasing the likelihood of a personal crisis, leading in some cases to self-harm or harm to others.

The report continued: "In turn, prejudices are reinforce and provoke even more coercise responses, resulting in a downward spiral, which we call 'circles of fear', in which staff see service users as potentially dangerous and service users perceive services as harmful."

- Ten key themes emerged from the research:
- There were circles of fear that stopped Black people from engaging with services.
- Mainstream services were experienced as inhumane, unhelpful and inappropriate. Black service users were not treated with respect and their voices were not heard. Services were not accessible, welcoming,

relevant or well integrated with the community.

- The care pathways of Black people were problematic and influenced the nature and outcome of treatment and the willingness of these communities to engage with mainstream services. Black people came to services too late, when they were already in crisis, reinforcing the circles of fear.
- Primary care involvement was limited and community-based crisis care was lacking.
- Acute care was perceived negatively and did not aid recovery.
- There was a divergence in professional and lay discourse on mental illness/distress. Different models and descriptions of mental illness were used and other people's philosophies or worldviews were not understood or even acknowledged.
- Service user, family and carer involvement was lacking.
- Conflict between professionals and service users was not always addressed in a beneficial way. The concept of 'culture' had been used in an attempt to address some of these issues, but had a tendency to divert professionals away from looking at individual histories, characteristics and needs.
- Black-led community initiatives were not valued. Specifically, secure funding and

long term capacity building initiatives were absent.
- Stigma and social inclusion were important dimensions in the lives of service users.

A wide ranging programme, addressed to both the statutory and Black communities, was identified as crucial to breaking the circles of fear. Its main aims were to ensure that Black service users were treated with respect and their voices heard; to deliver early intervention and early access to services to prevent escalation in crises; to make sure services were accessible, welcoming, relevant and well integrated with the community; to increase effective communication on both sides, including the creation of a culture allowing people to discuss race and mental health issues; and to deliver greater support and funding to services led by the Black community.

It was envisaged that the best way to realise these aims would be to empower the Black community to develop, or further develop, gateway organisations with the brief to build bridges between the community and services, and between individuals.

The report, according to its authors, represented a major step forward, "In turning this problem around and creating solutions that are owned and led by the Black community itself". In all, fifteen recommendations were made, of which, in the words of a spokesperson for the Sainsbury Centre

Crisis in the Community

for Mental Health, there has been, "Rather patchy implementation". These recommendations, and the Sainsbury Centre for Mental Health's view of the Government's response to each of them, were as follows:

- Gateway organisations should be commissioned to develop bridge-building programmes to support the reintegration of Black service users.
- "This isn't happening but there are Community Development Workers in place under *Delivering Race Equality in Mental Health,* and some trusts are investing in this. The voluntary sector needs much more support."
- A national resource centre must be developed to support the development of gateway organisations.
- "This hasn't happened either."
- The National Institute for Mental Health should create and fund a national programme of mental health promotion aimed at and owned by the Black community.
- "This hasn't been done."
- All health and social care communities with significant populations of Black people should identify practical steps to encourage early access in non-stigmatising or generic community settings as part of the National Service Framework for Mental Health implementation programmes.

- "This is happening in some places but, as with many of the recommendations, the result depends on where you live. Trusts such as Camden and Islington (in London) are doing this but others aren't."
- Advocacy for service users and support for carers needs to be available early in the cycle.
- "Again, this is happening in some places. Advocacy has now been included in the Mental Health Bill."
- Each health and social care community must ensure equal access to appropriate counselling and psychotherapy services.
- "This is not happening."
- Carers and advocates must be involved in care planning.
- "This is not happening, and care planning is patchy across the country anyway."
- Acute inpatient care for Black people must be sympathetically viewed.
- "This was also a recommendation of the subsequent David Bennett inquiry. Again, it depends on local trusts."
- Training programmes in mental health should be developed and implemented for the relevant generic workers. Specifically, Black primary care staff are a key resource in bridge building. They need to be appropriately trained, supported and developed.
- "Again, it varies from trust to trust. We have concerns about race equality training."

Crisis in the Community

- Staff development programmes must be implemented to support overall strategy. The national resource centre should act as a central point for information about training and development for NHS and gateway agency staff.
- "This one is more or less covered by *Delivering Race Equality*, which makes cultural awareness compulsory, but again, it varies from trust to trust."
- The leadership centre, part of the Department of Health's Modernisation Agency, should develop leadership programmes for Black staff in all relevant sectors, working with Black organisations and national partners.
- "This is not happening. The Modernisation Agency has ceased to exist and has been replaced by the Institute for Innovation and Improvement."
- The Government should create opportunities for local and national funding via mechanisms such as Section 64 (of the Health Services and Public Health Act 1968 - this gives the Secretary of State for Health power to make grants to voluntary organisations in England, whose activities support the Department of Health's policy objectives relating to health and personal social services) and neighbourhood renewal grants to Black organisations.

- "This is sort of happening. Section 64 funding is still going but not specifically directed."
- The development of a national voice for the Black user movement should be facilitated.
- "We didn't quite do this. The programme following *Breaking the Circles of Fear* was a national voice and facilitated networking. There are several networks running now, including The Afiya Trust, the BME Mental Health Network etc."
- The Department of Health should set relevant performance targets.
- "*Delivering Race Equality* has targets in it, but they might not be part of the performance management framework."
- The National Institute for Mental Health should develop a research strategy to evaluate and underpin the development of service solutions and community involvement.
- "There is lots of research going on, of varying kinds and with varying objectives." As the Sainsbury Centre for Mental Health spokesperson concluded, "Events overtake reports, particularly the Bennett inquiry findings in 2004. Our team did campaign for and work on *Delivering Race Equality* though, which wouldn't have been as radical without our work."

Crisis in the Community

Another report emerged a year after *Breaking the Circles of Fear,* this time from the National Institute of Mental Health in England. *Inside Outside: Improving Mental Health Services for Ethnic Minorities in England,* in the words of then Minister of State for Health, Jacqui Smith, marked the beginning of, "A historic dialogue". The Government, she said, was profoundly committed to race equality. "The testimony of many service users, carers and members of the Black and Minority Ethnic communities is that this aspiration is not yet a reality. I acknowledge this," Smith added. "Tackling ethnic inequalities within mental health services, in terms of prevention, early detection, access, diagnosis, care and quality of treatment and outcome is one of the greatest challenges facing us. We have an obligation to meet this challenge and tackle racism and institutional discrimination within our mental health services." Smith, some nine months before the publication of the *Independent Inquiry into the Death of David Bennett*, was using the kind of language John Reid would later disallow – "Racism and institutional discrimination within our mental health services".

The introduction to the report itself was even more damning of the disadvantage and discrimination that characterised the experiences of ethnic minority communities in England, "In almost all walks of life". It continued, "This is particularly true in the area of health and health care. People from Black and Minority Ethnic groups suffer from poorer health, have reduced life expectancy and have greater problems with access to health care than the majority White population. Over the years, there have been several policy and service initiatives within the National Health Service aimed at reducing ethnic variations in disease incidence, access to care and service experience. Mental health is an area of particular concern for the minority communities in this country. For decades, the disparities and inequalities between Black and Minority Ethnic groups and the majority White population in the rates of mental ill health, service experience and service outcome, have been the focus of concern, debate and much research. However, there is little evidence that such concerns have led to significant progress, either in terms of improvement in health status or a more benign service experience and positive outcome for Black and Minority Ethnic groups. If anything, the problems experienced by minority ethnic groups within our mental health services may be getting worse. At resent, there is no national strategy or policy specifically intended to improve either the mental health of minority ethnic groups or their care and treatment within mental health services. Previous approaches taken to address these problems have been either fragmented or selective. As a result, the 'ethnicity agenda' within mental health services has tended to become either marginalised or ignored. Although there have been significant policy and service development within mainstream mental health services over the last five years, national initiatives such as the Mental Health National Service Framework (MHNSF) and the NHS Plan for Mental Health do not adequately address the particular needs of Black and Minority Ethnic groups. The problems and challenges associated with ethnicity and mental health are complex and not amenable to either simple solutions or a single approach. Progress and change in this area is dependent on an inclusive process, involving politicians, policy makers, service providers from both statutory and voluntary sectors, service users and carers and most importantly, Black and Minority Ethnic communities themselves."

The problems of mental health care as experienced by Black and Minority Ethnic groups were identified as such:
- That there is an over-emphasis on institutional and coercive models of care.
- That professional and organisation requirements are given priority over individual needs and rights.
- That institutional racism exists within mental health care.

There again is that phrase "institutional racism"; the Government may find it contentious, but many of those working within the mental health sector have little difficulty acknowledging it as a matter of fact.

The report stated that in order to bring about change, in order to redress the balance which was tipped adversely against Black and Minority Ethnic service users, it was essential to place progressive community-based mental health at the centre of service development and delivery. Those who used mental health services had to be identified, first and foremost, as citizens with mental health needs, "Which are understood as located in a social and cultural context".

The marginality and social exclusion experienced by minority ethnic groups were significant in understanding the mental health experiences in these communities and their access to mental health services. The ethnic inequalities evident in most aspects of public life were likely to have a bearing on the mental health of Black and Minority Ethnic groups. Survey results appeared to confirm this. Psychiatric illness rates were generally higher in minority ethnic groups; they also experienced significant social adversity but had poorer social networks and support. There were ethnic differences in access to mental health services. Most tellingly, there were significant and sustained differences between the White majority and minority ethnic groups in experience of mental health services and the outcome of such service interventions. "There does not appear to be a single area of mental health care in this country in which Black and Minority Ethnic groups fare as well as, or better than, the majority White community," the report found. "Both in terms of service experience and the outcome of service interventions, they fare much worse than people from the ethnic majority do. In addition, disease burden associated with mental disorder appears to fall disproportionately on minority ethnic populations."

The focus for change envisaged by *Inside Outside* was two-fold: the current provisions of mental health care and the Black and Minority Ethnic communities themselves, the former requiring reappraisal of its policies and practices, the latter likely to benefit from investment in enhancing capability. This was based on three key initiatives for change, *inside*, within the services, and *outside*, within the communities.

The report concluded: "The NHS, mental health services in particular, service users and carers, voluntary and other non-Governmental organisations working within mental health, in partnership with Black and Minority Ethnic communities in this country, will have to take concerted
action in order to bring about specific change and improvement in mental health services, so that available services are not experienced as discriminatory or inappropriate. Action is needed at several levels - developing policy in relation to ethnicity and culture that is synergistic with the modernisation programme within mental health, making mental health interventions culturally congruent, improving the capabilities of the workforce, enhancing community capacity and raising awareness.

Specific and co-ordinated action is required to:

- Reduce and eliminate the current ethnic inequalities in mental health service experience and outcome.
- Develop the capabilities of the mental health workforce in providing appropriate and effective mental health services for a multicultural population.
- Invest in community development of minority ethnic groups aimed at achieving greater community participation and ownership around mental health."

Both *Breaking the Circles of Fear* and *Inside Outside* articulated Black and Minority Ethnic groups' largely negative experience of mental health. Both reports too recognised the institution of mental health as discriminatory, an institution where racial difference seemed to determine the quality of care administered. As illustrated in *Inside Outside,* "Cultural and racial stereotyping is a common experience in the context of assessment and decisions concerning treatment. This may well influence the types of services and diagnosis individuals from minority backgrounds seek and receive." And both reports outlined strategies for change, strategies which were laudable and indeed appeared practicable.

What became of *Inside Out* then? According to Jim Fowles, who heads up *Delivering Race Equality* at the Department of Health, it was superseded by the DRE action plan. "As DRE

Crisis in the Community

itself says, it reflects *Inside Out's* three key objectives – namely, reducing ethnic inequalities in the experience of mental health services, developing the cultural capability of services, and engaging with communities."

In 2003, the Department of Health published the consultation document *Delivering Race Equality: A Framework for Action.* This set out how those accountable for planning, delivering and monitoring local primary care and mental health services could improve services for users, relatives and carers from Black and Minority Ethnic communities. It asked for views on what needed to be done at national level to provide support and leadership to those carrying out this work.

John Reid, occupying the Health portfolio in another of his ministerial incarnations, spoke fine words about how essential it was to better the provision of services to Black and Minority Ethnic communities. "Ensuring that those communities are not only informed, but also willing and able to work in partnership with services, are not merely matters of fulfilling statutory obligations, important though those are. They are essential if we are to achieve our overall goals in modernising the health and social care system. While this holds true for all services, there has been particular concern for a number of years that adequate services and health outcomes have not been delivered to people from Black and Minority Ethnic communities experiencing mental illness and distress. There is clear evidence of the need to transform the services and outcomes experienced by these users and their relatives and carers. The current situation is unacceptable and unsustainable since it contradicts the basic value of equity that is a cornerstone of the NHS. It is no good us pretending to have these values and failing to recognise we need to change in order to live up to them. We cannot both support the NHS principle of equity and allow the existing situation to continue."

The framework would form the basis of the five-year action plan, *Delivering Race Equality in Mental Health Care,* the Government's response to the inquiry into the death of David Bennett. This was released in January 2005, more than a year after the inquiry findings were published. It took a loss of life in wholly avoidable circumstances to force the Government into confronting an issue that had been a constant source of concern within the African Caribbean community and within mental health for too long.

Crisis in the Community

Chapter Five

Dr Richard Stone's composure falters as he reels off the list of recommendations made by himself and his colleagues at the conclusion of the inquiry into the death of David Bennett. There is an almost imperceptible intake of breath as the former General practitioner and long-time anti-racism campaigner, arrested by his imagination of what Bennett had to endure in an 18-year battle against mental illness, of the "Black bastard" taunts that accentuated the young African Caribbean's desolate experience of psychiatric care, becomes overwhelmed. I am at first disconcerted by the tears, embarrassed for Dr Stone for allowing his humanity to get the better of him. It's not what you expect of someone whose unflappability, whose proficiency for judgement earned him a place not only on the Bennett inquiry panel, but also on the panel that oversaw the inquiry into the death of Stephen Lawrence. Then, as he wipes his eyes, I am embarrassed by my own uncomfortable reaction to the sight of a grown man crying, by the socially constructed aversion to displays of raw emotion, by my inability to see what Dr Stone sees – David Bennett as a boy, somebody's son, somebody's brother, somebody who suffered inside his head, somebody who suffered in the mental health system for nearly half his life. And somebody whose chances of emerging as a survivor were diminished by his African Caribbean origin.

David Burke

Dr Stone propounds a theory. It's about institutional racism and cigarette smoking in mental health services. "David Bennett socked a nurse, for reasons which could perhaps be justified if he were still alive to be asked. He knocked her out, and he died 25 minutes later, restrained face-down on the floor by five nurses. Every one of the five nurses who restrained David Bennett had been trained that restraint was to be used only as a last resort. They had all received training to use de-escalation techniques before restraint was considered, in order to prevent the need for restraint. They had all undergone training in how to reduce the high risk of death during restraint. None of them applied the de-escalation or restraint techniques they had been taught. Institutional racism is not a difficult concept. In demonstrating its corrosive and cumulative presence lays my one regret about my role in the Bennett inquiry. I did not appreciate until much later how significant was evidence about the implementation of the cigarette smoking policy at the Norvic Clinic. Cross-questioning of the nurses responsible for his care in Norwich confirmed that none of them expressed any racism against him. It also confirmed the determination of their anti-racism. However, David Bennett was subjected to repeated, unchecked racist abuse from other patients during his 18 years as a patient in Britain's mental health services. When asked about the racist abuse by other patients, his nurses told us they could not act to stop it because the other patients were also emotionally vulnerable. On hearing this reason for the third time, I asked them to tell me about the unit's policy on cigarette smoking. I was told the patients knew they could only smoke in the Quiet Room. I asked if they had difficulty enforcing the rule given the patients' emotional vulnerability, and was told that there was no real problem. Then the light dawned. Until then it had not even occurred to them that, if they could enforce rules about smoking with emotionally vulnerable patients, they could have and should have done the same with a ban on racist abuse. They vividly demonstrated what the Stephen Lawrence Inquiry defined as institutional racism – the kind of unwitting prejudice, ignorance, thoughtlessness and racial stereotyping which surely disadvantaged Black people such as David Bennett."

Dr Stone is convinced that the existence of a successful smoking policy, in the absence of any thought of how a policy on patient-on-patient racist abuse may be relevant to the care of Black patients, provides strong evidence for institutional racism.

"The almost entirely White-led staffing and management at the Norvic Clinic had not even realised that this abuse might affect the behaviour of Black patients. I do not believe that it was David Bennett's schizophrenia, or even the over-medication with anti-psychotic drugs, which led him to sock the nurse. The trigger was the revelation that the White patient had got off scot-free, while 'Rocky', had been punished by being transferred away from his room and his unit. David Bennett is dead.   We will never know whether or not it was the cumulative and corrosive effect of 18 years of unchallenged overt racism by other patients that led him to feel aggrieved that yet again it was he, the sole Black man around, who was given the higher penalty."

Dr Stone wants health ministers and the NHS Executive, "To order at once that patient-on-patient racist abuse is not tolerated", adding, "No matter how emotionally vulnerable the perpetrators may be, racist abuse can and must be challenged whenever it occurs, and Black patients must know that they will be supported if they are faced with it."

*

David Roy Bennett was born in Jamaica on 5 February 1960.   He arrived in England as an eight-year-old to join his family – mum, dad and eight siblings – who were living in Peterborough. His father was an engineer with the London Brick Company. At school the young David gained five CSE's. After finishing his education he worked as a signwriter for three years. This was his only job, health problems apparently truncating his career prospects.   David, a talented footballer, was offered a trainee post with a club shortly before his mental state deteriorated; but because of his illness he couldn't take it up. He was also an

Crisis in the Community

accomplished musician - the drums being a speciality - and a committed Rastafarian who set up a club for local devotees in Peterborough in 1980. This was the same year he began to show signs of poor mental health.

His sister, Dr Joanna Bennett, recalled, "David had problems with his behaviour and his emotions. He saw his General practitioner, who prescribed sleeping tablets for him but did not seem to be concerned about anything else. They did not work. We saw a spiritualist in London and that did not work. I took him to the local psychiatric unit at Peterborough General Hospital and he eventually saw the consultant psychiatrist, Dr Feggetter. Dr Feggetter was dismissive. He said that maybe it was cannabis intoxication. We took David home. We continued to take care of him."

David became paralysed down one side of his body and was eventually referred to The Gables, the psychiatric hospital ward at Peterborough General Hospital. "I again remember Dr Feggetter's attitude. He said David had some kind of mental illness which was induced by smoking marijuana. At that stage I do not remember anyone telling us David had schizophrenia. Mental illness is not something that the everyday person understands. Nobody explained anything to us. It would have been useful in those early days if somebody had just said, 'This is what is happening to him. This is what the family could do to help him'."

David Burke

Although his medical records for the 1980s are incomplete, David had at least two periods of in-patient treatment between 1980 and 1984. In November of the latter year, he was convicted of minor criminal offences. Before his sentencing, and at his solicitor's request, Dr Feggetter wrote a report to the court recommending that he be made subject to a probation order with the proviso that he received psychiatric treatment. Having been admitted to Peterborough District Hospital, he later discharged himself in a breach of his order. David was arrested and remanded in custody at HMP Bedford. When he returned to court, a further recommendation from Dr Feggetter that a probation order be issued with a condition of treatment was disregarded; David was sentenced to six months' imprisonment, the majority of which he served at HMP Stafford. Dr Bennett visited him there and was horrified by his appearance and behaviour. He was unwell and appeared to have been bullied by other inmates.

No positive diagnosis of schizophrenia had been made at this stage; indeed Dr Feggetter diagnosed David as suffering from cannabis-induced psychosis. The doctor was disinclined to diagnose schizophrenia because he found that the patient seemed to get better reasonably quickly with treatment by anti-psychotic drugs.
A month after his release from prison, David returned to The Gables. In July 1985, he was admitted to St Andrew's Hospital, Northampton, a

Crisis in the Community

private hospital with medium secure facilities, and a diagnosis of schizophrenia was finally confirmed. He was transferred to the Norvic Clinic in October. His mother, to whom he was very close, died later the same year.

In January 1986, David made the transition from the clinic to home in Peterborough, where he stayed for several months. He then stopped taking his medication and his mental health deteriorated. In December, he found himself re-admitted to St Andrew's Hospital for a medical report under Section 35 of the Mental Health Act 1983. He remained at St Andrew's until January in the following year; his tenure there was marred by some incidents of violence. He spent two days in Peterborough District Hospital but absconded twice and was deemed violent and unmanageable.

David spent several months at St Andrew's and later as an inpatient at Peterborough General Hospital. His illness became more severe. There were references in his medical notes to bizarre speech, threatening karate-like stances, mood swings and episodic violence. At Peterborough General he attacked a female nurse, kicking her in the chest and punching her, fracturing her ribs.

In April 1988, Dr Holding, a consultant psychiatrist at St Andrew's, referred David to Rampton Hospital, a high security institution, for consideration of admission. He stated, "With each succeeding episode of illness, both symptomatically and behaviourally, he has become more ill." Dr Murphy, a consultant psychiatrist at Rampton, was of the opinion that he didn't require treatment under conditions of maximum security. His schizophrenia, according to Dr Murphy, was exacerbated by a lack of co-operation with his treatment and supervision, and, on occasion, by his misuse of cannabis.

That same summer David had a council flat in the community and was supported by his hospital social worker. His sister, Dr Bennett, described this period as, "A circle of going into custody, being discharged to The Gables and then being discharged from there and then being re-admitted quickly again". She claimed that at St Andrew's David was, "Just drugged up. He told he was racially abused and that he was taunted and was not prepared to tolerate it. The community care he received primarily consisted of his injections. Nobody seemed concerned about what he did or did not do, where he was going with his life or whether he wanted a job, or whether he wanted any education or how the family was coping."

For the next four years, David was moved between St Andrew's, Peterborough District, The Gables and the Norvic Clinic. In 1993, considerable improvement in his mental state was noted. This was reflected in a letter to the Head of Nursing Services at the Norvic Clinic in which he articulated his concerns. David wrote, "As you

Crisis in the Community

know, there are over half a dozen Black boys in this clinic. I don't know if you have realised that there are no Africans on your staff at the moment. We feel there should be at least two Black persons in the medical or social work staff. For the obvious reasons of security and contentment for all concerned, please do your best to remedy this appalling situation."

The reply indicated that there had been no application by any Black person to join the staff for the previous two and a half years.

The relative calm of 1994 was disrupted again the next year when he absconded from The Gables and had an altercation with one of his brothers. In August, he was sent to Heron Lodge at Hellesdon Hospital near Norwich. His condition deteriorated, and in one instance he threw a knife at a member of the nursing staff.

His admission to the Norvic Clinic in October 1995 was notable for his co-operation. But records showed him to be noticeably thought-disordered; there was loosening of associations and neologisms, he had paranoid ideas and delusions of ability, he was experiencing auditory hallucinations and had no insight into his condition.

In January 1996, David was subjected to an assault by a fellow patient, who also racially abused him. There was no record of any action being taken as a result of either the assault or the abuse.

He was transferred from Thorpe Ward at the Norvic Clinic to the less intensive, rehabilitative Drayton Ward. But a violent incident, in which members of the nursing staff received minor injuries and David had to be physically restrained, led to his return to Thorpe Ward in February.

During the first six months of 1986, he visited his sister, Winifred Bennett, in Peterborough on several occasions. He also saw his father – who by then was battling lung cancer – in July. When Mr Bennett died in August, despite initial hesitation from both medical authorities at the Norvic Clinic and his family, it was decided that David should attend the funeral. He did so without incident.

In October, there was a scene with a female taxi driver. He verbally abused her and then caused damage to her car, before assaulting a member of the Norvic Clinic nursing staff who had intervened in an effort to sort out the problem.

Dr Bennett phoned Thorpe Ward in November in response to a conversation she'd had with David during which he'd complained of being over-medicated. The inquiry report into his death noted that his, "Reluctance to take medication was the subject of fairly frequent entries in the records".

*

Crisis in the Community

Dr Feggetter, the consultant psychiatrist who first treated David at Peterborough District Hospital in 1980, told the Bennett inquiry panel that David was, "A nice young man who kept his personality and did not lose it as chronic schizophrenic patients tend to do". He had a sense of humour and, when he was well, managed well for himself. But Dr Feggetter also found David troublesome.

Dr Sagovsky, who took over David's care from Dr Feggetter in 1990, agreed that he wasn't always easy to work with because of his dislike of authority of any description. If he had the sense that anyone was not treating him as an equal or almost as a friend he would not, "Take anything from them".

His propensity for violence, combined with his athleticism, meant staff were quite frightened of David. But Dr Sagovsky acknowledged he had charm. "He was a lovely bloke but quite a handful," she said. Other African Caribbean patients looked up to him - he was their "mascot".

David had difficulty in accepting support. He was quick to feel patronised and didn't like boundaries. On occasions when he went to see Dr Sagovsky he would want to put his arm around her and call her Ruth.

She recalled that, at times, the levels of medication David was prescribed were higher than almost any patient she'd known. He was sometimes on as many as three anti-psychotic drugs concurrently.

The inquiry panel, reviewing the history of David's mental illness and the treatment he received, concluded from the evidence presented that there wasn't any real attempt to engage his family in the management of his condition from 1980 to 1998. The report states: "There is no indication that his racial, cultural or social needs were adequately attended to. The general impression throughout this lengthy period is of a man who was treated at times with consideration by individual nurses, at times with a degree of intolerance and at times as if he were a nuisance who had to be contained. The notes at St Andrew's, Northampton, in the 1980s, particularly give the impression that he was often considered a nuisance and was given heavy doses of anti-psychotic drugs to contain him. No secret was made of his medication. His notes were regularly seen by various psychiatrists at various institutions. But there is no indication that any doctor at any institution commented that the amount of drugs he was getting at the time was unusual or too high."

*

Dr Stanley began work as a consultant psychiatrist at the Norvic Clinic in January 1998, and was immediately appointed David's responsible medical officer. She devised an individualised care plan for her new charge. David had the

Crisis in the Community

opportunity to listen to music and to watch television of his choice. He was taken regularly to Carrow Road football ground to watch Norwich City. Mindful that he was a practicing Rastafarian, Dr Stanley allowed David space to put up posters and wear clothes relating to his faith. He went on community trips with the staff and visited his family regularly.

Her considered opinion was that he suffered from hebephrenic schizophrenia, a form of schizophrenia characterised by a severe disintegration of personality, including erratic speech, childish mannerisms and bizarre behaviour. Dr Stanley reckoned the most suitable medication for this condition was Clozapine, the dosage of which was increased as David's mental state worsened. She went on leave in October 1998, by which time David was on 650mg of the drug per day. The maximum British National Formulary dose then was 900mg per day as a long-term option. Dr Stanley recalled that David required intensive nursing intervention, he was unpredictable, and his stay at the Norvic Clinic had exceeded what was initially anticipated. During much of 1998 he was slowly continuing to deteriorate.

David was not referred for psychological treatment because Dr Sedgwick, the psychologist responsible for him in the last year of his life, felt he wasn't well enough for such intervention.

David Burke

David Bennett was formally pronounced dead at the Nofolk & Norwich Hospital at 0020 hours on 31 October 1998. But he had actually died some time earlier at the Norvic Clinic medium secure unit.

David had spent the day of 30 October on Drayton Ward. His key worker, Mr Ncube, saw him periodically; he didn't notice anything untoward taking place, nor did David behave in an unusual or inappropriate way. When Mr Ncube went off duty at 2105 hours, he spoke to David before leaving and reported that he appeared to be fine.

At about 2200 hours, a patient – known as DW - was using the one telephone on Drayton Ward to call his mother. He had been on the phone for between 45 and 60 seconds when David asked him how long he was going to be. David then left and returned later. He seemed angry and told DW, "Give me the fucking phone." DW told him to go away; David grabbed the phone out of DW's hand, and he in turn retrieved it. Then David threw a punch; his hand hit the phone, which then struck DW's face. It was quite a hard blow; there was blood.

Shortly after being hit, DW went to David's bedroom, kicked on his door and shouted at him. He was extremely offensive and racist in his remarks. Evidence presented at the inquiry indicated that he called David "a Black bastard", and said, "You niggers are all the same." David opened the door and was punched on the chin by DW.

Nursing Assistant Bartlett was the first member of staff on the scene. He saw David emerge from his bedroom, at which point he and DW started to fight. DW was using his fists while David was trying to karate kick DW. By the time DW punched David in the jaw; two other nurses arrived, grabbed hold of DW and took him away from David. DW was still uttering obscenities and racist remarks.

One of the nurses suggested that David went to his room. He complied but was clearly agitated. David washed his mouth, which was bleeding. Nursing Assistant Bartlett asked if he could have a look but David refused. He said nobody cared for him and he had nothing to look forward to. David then made reference to DW and said he was, "Going to fucking kill him". He asked Nursing Assistant Bartlett to leave his room, which he did. David followed him as he walked towards the area of the ward to which DW had gone, saying repeatedly that he was going to kill him. Nursing Assistant Bartlett tried to calm David down to prevent another incident between the two men. DW was taken to his bedroom by other members of staff to avoid any further confrontation. David sat on a chair in Drayton Ward's day area.

Staff Nurse Deeks telephoned Thorpe Ward and asked Staff Nurse Fixter if it would be possible for David to stay in that ward overnight; he judged

David's mental state to be fragile, and didn't think it appropriate to transfer DW to Thorpe Ward because his mental state was not an issue. Before arranging his transfer, Staff Nurse Deeks gave David his medication, which he took without any difficulty.

As David was being taken to Thorpe Ward, he said, "I don't know why it's me that's going." Staff Nurse Deeks replied, "Well, you need to." It was around 2255 hours. Staff Nurse Deeks intended to talk to DW about the racist abuse, but in view of what then happened, "events took over".

On his arrival in Thorpe Ward, David proceeded to roll a cigarette and his mood was calmer. Staff Nurse Hadley told him he was going to stay the night on the ward. David replied, "Yep, yep, OK." Then he asked, "What about DW?" Staff Nurse Hadley was in the process of answering that DW was staying on Drayton when David punched her on the left side of her face at least three times. The first punch knocked her backwards and she tried to block the other punches, shielding her face with her arms. She didn't remember falling to the ground but remembered being on the ground and being dragged away by another patient. Her vision was blurred as a result of the blow. She felt very hot and dizzy, and was very scared.

Nursing Assistant Clapham, who saw David hit Staff Nurse Hadley, described the violence as, "Just horrendous". He and Staff Nurse Fixter

Crisis in the Community

attempted to restrain David. Nursing Assistant Clapham had hold of his right arm; all three men went to the floor. David seized Nursing Assistant Farrow's jumper near her neck and began to twist it. She gagged and shouted, "He is strangling me", before falling to the floor with the others. Nursing Assistant Clapham used a thumb lock to release David's hand. He was urging David to calm down, while David was shouting, "God doesn't love me, the devil is after me. They're trying to kill me."

According to Staff Nurse Fixter, Staff Nurse Robson and Student Nurse Moore were assisting in trying to placate David; but he couldn't say precisely where they were as he had his back to them. He thought they were on David's legs.

It was after an ambulance carrying Staff Nurse Hadley had left that Staff Nurse Fixter realised David had gone quiet. He took David's blood pressure, which read 120/60. Staff Nurse Fixter said it wasn't possible on that night for a nurse to have hold of David's head, so there was no nurse in that position. This would have been the correct procedure in role play, but in a live situation, when dealing with someone of an extremely psychotic nature, it didn't work. Even when David was pinned to the ground, his body was still bucking up and down.

There came a time when Staff Nurse Fixter instructed all physical restraints to be lifted. He took a wrist pulse, which was very weak. He could not detect a radial pulse. Later he contradicted himself and said that he found no pulse. Staff Nurse Fixter turned David on his right side in the recovery position and cleared his airway before attempting cardiac resuscitation. Oxygen was brought in and Staff Nurse Fixter applied four litres through the face mask. This had no effect. By the time an ambulance had been summoned to take David to hospital, he had been apparently unconscious for about ten minutes. The paramedics applied defibrillation devices without success. They used an ambi-bag and Staff Nurse Fixter performed chest compression. David was placed on a stretcher. A paramedic informed Staff Nurse Fixter that, in his view, David was dead. He was removed to the Norfolk & Norwich Hospital, accompanied by Nursing Assistant Clapham and Staff Nurse Evans.

*

Staff Nurse Fixter felt that on that evening there was a shortage of staff, a shortage of medical cover and no adequate response team on duty at the Norvic Clinic. The appropriate number of staff should have been four. There were, in fact, four nurses on Thorpe Ward at the time of the incident, but Staff Nurse Fixter still maintained he was short staffed in terms of patient/staff ratio.

Crisis in the Community

He was unable to obtain an approved lock on David's left arm during the violent struggle; he never leant on his chest or his shoulder. As far as Staff Nurse Fixter was aware, David's legs were being pinned by Staff Nurse Robson and Nursing Assistant Marris. He believed they were across David's buttocks - just below his buttocks and ankles – just securing him to prevent movement.

Nursing Assistant Clapham had a good relationship with David. He used to take him to see Winifred in Peterborough regularly and they played football together. When David was well he was "a super lad"; but when he was ill he could be nasty and intimidating.

Having trained in control and restraint, Nursing Assistant Clapham explained, "If you are restraining somebody, first and foremost you have to make sure they are comfortable while you are restraining them, because it's not a nice thing being held down on the floor."

On the evening of 30 October, while being restrained, David was talking to Nursing Assistant Clapham constantly about football and anything else that came into his mind. "I wanted the boy to be as calm as can be before I am prepared to let him up," Nursing Assistant Clapham said. He had hold of David's right arm and Staff Nurse Fixter was holding his left arm. Nursing Assistant Clapham lay on the floor by David's right side, but was not lying on him; he put his right leg across the bottom of his legs as he was still thrashing around. The idea was not to restrain patients on the floor, but this was the only course of action in this instance to keep David calm.

Nursing Assistant Clapham said that when it came to restraining patients as violent as David, "the classroom stuff" could be thrown out the window. The female nurses were on his legs and he was still thrashing up and down. Nobody was holding his head because his head was in a comfortable position.

When Nursing Assistant Clapham returned to the Norvic Clinic from the Norfolk & Norwick Hospital at around 0130 hours, the police were there. They refused to let him go home, warning that they would lock him up for the night if he didn't stay. The police wanted his clothes for forensic testing; Nursing Assistant Clapham felt he was being treated like a criminal. The police wouldn't allow staff to discuss the incident in the hours after David's death. "Regardless of what the boy has done, that's still someone who has died in my arms and that is a hard thing to live with," he said.

*

Nursing Assistant Marris and Student Nurse Moore were alerted at 2254 hours to go from Drayton Ward, where they were on duty, to Thorpe Ward. They found Staff Nurse Hadley on the floor with staff who were struggling with David.

Crisis in the Community

Nursing Assistant Marris lay across David's legs and secured his ankles. She recollected seeing Staff Nurse Robson lying across his buttocks. As Nursing Assistant Marris lay down, David kicked her in the ribs. He was shouting, "They are going to kill me, get them off, they are going to kill me". At some stage Student Nurse Moore got up and was replaced by Nursing Assistant Farrow. Eventually David ceased struggling.

After being relieved by Nursing Assistant Farrow, Student Nurse Moore went to fetch Staff Nurse Hadley's personal possessions from Eton Ward. When she returned to Thorpe Ward, David was still being restrained by Staff Nurse Fixter, and Nursing Assistants Clapham, Farrow and Marris. There came a point when, once he had calmed down, they rolled him over. She saw he was incontinent of urine. Student Nurse Moore detected a faint pulse in both his wrist and neck and Staff Nurse Fixter checked his blood pressure before placing him in the recovery position.

When oxygen was administered to David, the nursing staff realised he was not breathing. Staff Nurses Fixter and Evans then administered cardio-pulmonary resuscitation. The paramedics came and took him away on a trolley. Student Nurse Moore wasn't able to remember precisely where Staff Nurse Robson was in relation to David's body, but thought that she was next to her, higher up. They had not been taught to restrain a patient by having two or three person on their legs, but were in a situation where one person could not adequately restrain David from using his legs.

Nursing Assistant Farrow never heard Staff Nurse Fixter issuing instructions to anybody about the holds they should be using until he asked them all to release their holds. He did not tell people how to restrain David.

Mr Holdsworth was an ambulance paramedic who, along with his colleagues, went to the Norvic Clinic upon receiving an emergency message that a female member of staff had been assaulted. As they entered Thorpe Ward, he noticed a person lying on the floor, face down. He could see four people attending to the person, two females lying on their fronts over the person's legs, one male lying over the person's upper torso with his body on the far side of the person and a fourth person, a male, by the person's head. The person on the floor – David - did not appear to be struggling.

Mrs Chambers, general manager of the Norvic Clinic, had the responsibility for the management and co-ordination of the nursing and administrative staff. She was at home but on call on the evening of 30 October. At 2305 hours, a telephone call informed her there had been an incident in which a member of staff had been hurt. She immediately went to the clinic.

Crisis in the Community

Mrs Chambers was about to accompany Staff Nurse Hadley to the hospital when, concerned about David, she looked across to where he was being restrained. He wasn't struggling but was motionless. The nurses were talking to him. She saw Staff Nurse Fixter by David's head, holding one of his arms. Everything seemed to be under control, otherwise, Mrs Chambers said, she would not have gone to the hospital with Staff Nurse Hadley.

DS, a patient in Thorpe Ward, said David did not get on with Staff Nurse Fixter. "They had their ups and downs," was how he put it. He remembered David being, "Sort of struggled onto the floor" and restrained by his throat, to which pressure was being applied. DS heard David say, "Get off me, get off me, I can't breathe. Get off my throat." Staff Nurse Fixter had his hand round David's throat and wasn't applying pressure to any other part of his body.

Another patient, GH, summarised the assault on Staff Nurse Hadley as follows: "One of the nurses from another ward came over and spoke to 'Rocky'. 'Rocky' jumped up and hit her in the jaw; the force of the blow threw the nurse up against the radiator. Both I and another patient tried to help the nurse. Several nurses came into the room. Bruce Fixter told us all to go to bed. Bruce and two lady nurses held 'Rocky' on the floor. Bruce was lying across 'Rocky's' legs. 'Rocky' was rolling around on the floor struggling, trying to get away and saying, 'They are trying to kill me'. I did not see anything wrong with the way the nurses were dealing with 'Rocky'."

When it was established that David had collapsed and was not responding by either word of mouth or by actions, Staff Nurse Fixter took his blood pressure and then his wrist pulse. He turned David into the recovery position, and examined his airways, ensuring they were clear. David was then laid on his back, his head supported by a rolled up blanket. Staff Nurse Fixter shone a torch into his eyes but couldn't see any reaction. At some stage Nursing Assistant Mariss said she thought David had stopped breathing.

A joint decision was made to conduct cardio-pulmonary resuscitation. Staff Nurse Fixter carried out mouth-to-mouth resuscitation while Staff Nurse Evans compressed the chest at a 5-1 ratio. There were slight signs that David was breathing. Four litres of oxygen were pumped through an oxygen face mask, with no result. Some ten minutes had elapsed since the staff first became worried about David. An ambulance had been summoned at this stage.

The ambulance arrived at 2345 hours. The paramedics applied a defibrillator to David's chest. They operated it for about five minutes, with no result. An Ambi bag was then used, again without success. Mr Rogers, one of the paramedics,

Crisis in the Community

observing stiffness in the arms suggestive of rigor
mortis, formed the view that David was dead.

Chapter Six

The panel which oversaw the inquiry into the death of David Bennett comprised Professor David Sallah, a professor of mental health, Professor Sashi Sashidharan, a consultant psychiatrist, Dr Richard Stone, a former general practitioner, Joyce Struthers, a Community Health Council member and former chair of the Association of Community Health Councils of England and Wales and Sir John Blofeld, a retired High Court judge.

The evidence they heard during the inquiry raised a number of issues which were considered by the panel. These included racism at the Norvic Clinic, the decision to move David to Thorpe Ward, medication, control and restraint, emergency procedures, the medical presence at the clinic, staff attitudes to David, the failure to inform the family of his death and the post mortem results.

The panel was unable to find any evidence of deliberate racism at the clinic. There were no instances of racist abuse directed at David by members of staff, though there were instances of racist abuse by other patients. The inquiry report stated: "The evidence we have heard, together with our own experience, leads us to the conclusion that racist abuse is highly insidious. Where there is racist abuse it inevitably has an effect upon its victim. The victim is bound to feel acutely sensitive and frequently has the desire to retaliate, particularly if their perception is that no action may be taken to prevent racist abuse." However, it was pointed out that the local nursing staff were recruited locally and were predominantly White. The vast majority of patients were also White. Dr Shetty, a consultant psychiatrist at the clinic, warned, "There is a risk that, in places like Norwich, people may never develop the awareness and skills to deal with Black people because there are so few of them."

Dr Solomka, another consultant psychiatrist at the clinic, said there were very limited facilities for Black and Minority Ethnic groups in the Norwich area, especially for African Caribbeans. There were no clubs, no advocacy groups and no recreational activities.

Insufficient attention was paid to David's cultural, social and religious needs, and not enough effort was made to recruit Black and Minority Ethnic staff.

The panel felt the decision to move David from Drayton Ward to Thorpe Ward was handled, "With insufficient care and sensitivity". The report went on: "We accept that David Bennett acted inappropriately in trying to persuade the patient DW to let him use the telephone and was at fault in punching him when he refused to do so. But the reaction of DW by using violence accompanied by repeated racist abuse inevitably left David Bennett feeling that he was the injured party. The failure by staff to take up the issue of racist abuse before either patient was removed from Drayton Ward was regrettable. Nurses had the opportunity to talk to both patients at that stage. When the decision was made to move David Bennett to Thorpe Ward, David Bennett, by his words and actions, showed that he considered that it was taken because he was a Black man and DW was White. No attempt was made to explain to David Bennett that this was not the case. We have formed the strong and disturbing view that the issue of race was not taken into account when this decision was taken to move David Bennett to Thorpe Ward."

The panel concluded that the staff didn't appreciate the need to speak to either patient in an attempt to de-escalate the incident. They didn't appreciate the importance of doing this because, "They were unaware of the corrosive and cumulative effect of racist abuse upon a Black patient". The decision to remove David was bound to have left him with the overwhelming feeling that he had been wrongly criticised and wrongly removed from Drayton Ward.

Furthermore, the panel was of the impression that on the evening of his death David was not treated by the nurses as if he were capable of being talked to like a rational human being, but was in fact treated as if he were "a lesser being" who should be ordered about and not be given the opportunity to articulate his own views about the decision before a decision was made.

Dr Lipsedge, a consultant psychiatrist, was asked by the Bennett family's solicitors to consider expert reports from witnesses called at the inquest into David's death in relation to the issue of control and restraint. He said, "Trying to subdue a violently struggling patient is not only a dreadful experience for the patient, but it is also dreadful for the staff, for the nurses and for the doctors. And the longer it goes on the worse that ordeal is in terms of psychological stress to the whole team and to the patient and indeed to the relatives and to the other patients and everybody who might witness it. So there are very good reasons, if you like, non-medical reasons, reasons to do with the humane approach to patients, to try and get to limit the period of restraint as much as possible."

The inquiry felt it was negligent not to have a nurse taking proper control of David's head throughout the incident. Once David was on the floor, Staff Nurse Fixter – as the senior nurse on Thorpe Ward – should have either moved to the head himself or instructed one of the other nurses to do so.

The report continued: "The training that he had received clearly indicated that the nurse at the head is the number one nurse in charge. In view of the fact that there were only two male nurses involved, it might have been difficult for Staff

.

Nurse Fixter to have relinquished his hold on David Bennett's arm so that he could move to the head. That does not excuse his failure to ensure that some other nurse was at his head. If that had been done, we consider that signs of distress would have been detected earlier than they were and that there was a real possibility that this death might never have occurred."

Restraint was mishandled by the nursing staff. There were nurses pressing onto David's body when they should not have been; as a consequence, his capacity to breathe adequately was restricted so that he was unable to inhale sufficient oxygen. "We also conclude that the restraint continued for substantially longer than was safe. We recognise that the training in control and restraint given to the staff at the Norvic Clinic at that time put no limit on the time that a patient could be restrained in the prone position, so we do not make any criticism of the nursing staff about this, but we regard it as a serious failure of training."
The evidence indicated that the nurses should have attempted to resuscitate David sooner. This would have been more likely had there been a nurse at his head, in a position to observe that David had not simply stopped struggling but was in a state of collapse.

A catalogue of human error meant that Dr Bishram, the duty doctor who covered the Norvic Clinic, didn't arrive until just before midnight –

some one hour and fifteen minutes after he was called. If Dr Bishram had been present shortly after being first asked to attend, he may have been able to save David's life. According to the report: "He could have monitored the nurses' use of restraint. Alternatively, he could have asked them to move David Bennett to the seclusion room or he could have administered an intravenous injection of tranquillising medicine."

On the issue of staff attitudes to David, the panel couldn't find any detailed assessment of his overall ethnic needs; these were occasionally addressed by individual sympathetic nurses who looked after him. "We find no coherent pattern or plan for the treatment of these highly important needs, nor do we find any pattern of engaging members of his family in the problems that faced him. We note that he was seen by numerous different doctors and nurses in the various hospitals he attended, many of whom had had experience in other parts of the country where there are more patients from the Black and Minority Ethnic communities. But there was no evidence that any of them suggested any alteration in the way David Bennett's ethnic needs were met or made any criticism of his existing regime of treatment. This leads us to suppose that the treatment received by David Bennett, as an African Caribbean, is likely to have been the same as the treatment received by other patients from the Black and Minority Ethnic communities with similar health problems. They too are likely to

David Burke

have spent lengthy periods in locked wards or
hospitals and to have been treated with high
doses of anti-psychotic medication. These failures
contributed to David Bennett's problems. We do
not go so far as to suggest that, without them, his
mental health problems would have been radically
alleviated, but we are left in no doubt that they
seriously diminished the quality of his life."

Mrs Chambers, general manager of the Norvic
Clinic, reported David's death to police at 0040
hours on 31 October from the accident and
emergency department at the Norfolk and Norwich
Hospital. Staff at the Norvic Clinic were told by
police not to contact David's family, that they
would arrange for it to be done. David's sister,
Winifred, was first informed of the tragic news by
police at 0900 hours. Later, she spoke to a
clinical nurse specialist but failed to establish what
had happened to her brother. There was no
further communication between the Norvic Clinic
and the Bennett family for the remainder of the
weekend, except to arrange a meeting on the
Monday.

The meeting ended in disorder after Dr Stanley
was unable to answer questions about David's
death in detail. To allow the Bennetts to leave the
meeting without a reasonably full disclosure of the
relevant facts was, "Not only inhumane but also
bound to lead the family to suspect that there was
some cover-up going on".

Crisis in the Community

The subsequent post-mortem was carried out by Dr Harrison, a consultant pathologist and Dr Cary, the consultant pathologist appointed by the Bennett family. Both concurred that there was evidence of superficial and deep bruising at autopsy, but no evidence of fractures or assault-type injuries.

Dr Harrison identified restraint in the prone position for a length of time as the most important factor leading to death. He said, "I understand that restraint in that position can be carried out relatively safely, although some people say you should never restrain in the prone position; but the time interval is critical. In this case I understand it was 15 to 20 minutes, which I think was far too long."

Chapter Seven

While people from all communities found it difficult to access mental health services, those from the Black and Minority Ethnic communities found it especially so, according to the *Independent Inquiry into the Death of David Bennett.*

A further problem concerned the initial diagnosis in a patient. Psychiatrists sometimes made a diagnosis of drug-induced psychosis, which, when it came to African Caribbeans, nearly always related to the use of cannabis. There appeared to be no clear medical basis for this diagnosis and indeed indications were that it prohibited proper treatment of early signs of schizophrenia.

As pointed out in the *Breaking the Circles of Fear* report, the Black and Minority Ethnic community feared that if they engaged with mental health services they would be locked up for a long time, if not for life and treated with medication that could eventually kill them. Young Black men with signs of mental illness frequently, again out of fear, did not go to their doctor until the illness was so pronounced that family and friends could no longer cope.

There was over-representation in Black people failing to respond to treatment for schizophrenia; they tended to receive higher doses of anti-psychotic mediation than White people with similar health problems; they were generally regarded by

Crisis in the Community

mental health staff as more aggressive, more alarming, more dangerous and more difficult to treat; and instead of being discharged back into the community, they were more likely to remain as long-term patients.

Adopting the definition of institutional racism as outlined by Sir William Macpherson in *the Stephen Lawrence Inquiry,* the Bennett inquiry found that some people failed to understand it, while others didn't appreciate that it was the culmination of unwitting prejudice, ignorance, thoughtlessness or racial stereotyping. Rather they considered that institutional racism was deliberate – a misconception that needed to be addressed.

The representatives of Mind who gave evidence to the inquiry were in no doubt that institutional racism existed within the NHS and that it meant "a heart-and-mind attitude to Black people". There was a lack of awareness of cultural issues, of how people came from within their communities, and of their values and aspirations.

Errol Francis of the Sainsbury Centre for Mental Health, and co-author of *Breaking the Circles of Fear*, regarded the use of the word "racism" as unhelpful. Instead, he said, it was necessary to deconstruct what racism was about – namely, human relationships based on power, the power of one person over another. He emphasised that Black patients were particularly sensitive to any hint of regulation, control or disrespect because they had been primed by their experiences to expect to be treated badly in society.

Dr Joanna Bennett felt there should be greater focus on how practitioners were enabled in dealing with people as people. Taking time to find out what really mattered to a person was more important than talking about culture, ethnicity and cultural competence. A better understanding of the ideology of racism, and how it created stereotypes, assumptions and values, was also imperative.

Professor Kevin Gournay of King's College at the University of London was of the opinion that not enough was being done to train nurses and doctors to appreciate the issue of culture and the way people manifested their mental health problems. If they were not trained until they qualified and had been doing their jobs for two or three years, their attitudes and experiences were entrenched; they already saw Black patients, for example, as potential crack dealers and a source of violent incidents. At this stage it was too late to do anything about training; it had to be done earlier.

Alicia Spence, manager of the African Caribbean Cultural Initiative based in Wolverhampton, told the inquiry that mental health services were almost devoid of humanity. When Black people presented themselves, they may be talking louder

Crisis in the Community

than normal, or gesticulating; but mental health symptoms were often misunderstood and misinterpreted because, when faced with a Black person, the professionals were expecting trouble. It followed that their response was sometimes inappropriate. It was essential, Spence continued, to have an understanding of other people's culture and their mannerisms. Language was a major issue too. When under strain, people reverted to their mother tongue. If healthcare professionals didn't understand fully what they were saying, there was room for misinterpretation and misunderstanding. On some occasions an interpreter may be needed.

Consultant psychiatrist Dr Stephen Pereira wanted a zero tolerance approach to racist abuse between patients. Dr Maurice Lipsedge, emeritus consultant psychiatrist, suggested that if there was a climate on the ward in a psychiatric unit where profoundly damaging expressions of racism were disregarded by staff or given low priority, the patients with racist attitudes would deem it was alright to express them. The victims would consequently feel unsupported, devalued, dehumanised and objectified. He wished to see vivid written notices in each ward that racist language was not permitted.

Dr Chandra Ghost, a consultant forensic psychiatrist, emphasised that the young Black men who ended up in secure facilities were Black British. Their needs were quite different from what might have been the difficulties or cultural needs of their grandparents or great-grandparents. He proposed more training for all concerned into the various problems and facets of racism. That training programme should include the history of Black immigration and Black slavery.

The inquiry heard convincing evidence that there was too little contact with the family of the patient by those entrusted with treatment and care. Family contacts and family involvement were vital if the patient was to be successfully treated in the community; when a patient was in a mental health hospital, this contact should still be maintained.

Dr Bennett claimed there was insufficient involvement with David's family by mental health services during the many years of his illness. The family could easily have helped if they had been made aware of such things as the provision of clothing, money and advice on culture and social issues. She also spoke about the lack of communication from the mental health services about the treatment he was receiving. Once a patient was in the system, the family were largely ignored.

Dr Ghosh said that staff, when dealing with Black patients, perceived families as a nuisance. Black mothers were regarded as highly problematic. There was not only an attempt by staff not to give them information, but there was a feeling of hostility towards the families.

*

The evidence about medication in cases of schizophrenia led the inquiry to strongly recommend an urgent need for further research and investigation into the subject by Government agencies and other relevant organisations, including the Royal Colleges. The views of patients should form an important part of these investigations.

Dr Bennett said this had to be looked at in the context of over-medication of Black patients. There had to be clearer guidance about administering more than one type of anti-psychotic drug at any one time. She also urged research on the link between anti-psychotic drugs and their possible adverse effects on one patient in the case of that patient having to be physically restrained.

Professor Louis Appleby, national director for mental health, indicated there was widespread suspicion that in clinical care young people from the Black community tended to be given higher doses of individual anti-psychotic drugs or poly-medication because they were perceived by the staff to be more dangerous or more of a nuisance. But it was not something that had been picked up in research; therefore, more research was necessary.

*

The inquiry learned that the behaviour of people suffering from mental illness may occasionally be difficult for their practitioners to deal with; this challenging behaviour required a sensitive and sympathetic attitude, with prevention being the preferred course of action. It was acknowledged that this was not always possible, in which case de-escalation should be attempted. This could be done in many ways: by talking with the patient, by moving the patient to different surroundings; or, where there was an argument between two or more patients, by separating them firmly but gently. In a few instances neither prevention nor de-escalation were viable, whereby oral medication, for the purposes of sedation, may be required. If medication didn't work, or was for some reason inappropriate, the other alternatives were restraint or seclusion.

The Royal College of Nursing commented that control and restraint was used too early on patients, especially Black and Minority Ethnic patients. Once hands were laid on the patient, a threatening situation was likely to become a violent one. Professor Appleby advocated restraint only as a last resort. It should be seen as a therapeutic process following strict guidelines. Errol Francis described as "crude" the idea of meeting force with force in a medical environment. It was vital that staff were more familiar with the whole psychology of the relationships between patients and staff. They had to understand what turned people violent and how to defuse a violent situation.

The inquiry panel formed a firm view that it was not apposite to inflict deliberate pain during the restraint of a patient, whatever the circumstances. Any patient requiring physical restraint was, by definition, in a medical emergency.

Dr Nat Cary, who carried out a post-mortem on David at the Bennett family's request, considered that there were times when a very carefully applied painful hold could be the most humane way of dealing with a person.

The inquiry was convinced that it was always dangerous to place a person in a facedown prone position, but accepted there were occasions when there was no alternative. It was opposed to mechanical restraints because of the ambiguity surrounding their effectiveness; they were also seen as degrading and were open to abuse.

Whenever a mentally ill patient was detained, there should be a fully-equipped resuscitation trolley and people trained in the use of the equipment, available at all times. A doctor should be present or, if that wasn't possible, foolproof arrangements should be in place to guarantee a doctor's attendance within twenty minutes of a request by staff to do so.

*

The inquiry concluded on a cautionary note. A number of initiatives had been instigated in the preceding years by the Department of Health; while each had been well-intentioned and had performed useful work, management changes had resulted in a loss of impetus. "There have been many conferences, consultations and papers written during the last twenty years about the problems that the mental health services face. Some of these have dealt with the problems experienced by the Black and Minority Ethnic communities. Time and again regrets at the existing state of affairs have been expressed. While it would be unfair to say that nothing has happened, it is true to say that not very much and certainly not enough has happened. Unless there are sufficient resources and sustained management, which is both dedicated and committed, these problems cannot be solved," the inquiry report stated. "At present, people from the Black and Minority Ethnic communities involved in the mental health services are not getting the service they are entitled to. Putting it bluntly, this is a disgrace. The NHS is national. Final responsibility lies fairly and squarely with the Department of Health. Other institutions may advise and may contribute to what should be done. But, individually or collectively, they have little power to require that changes be made. We are told that the Department of Health is determined to carry out the necessary improvements. We very much hope that this time they will. But, in view of the history, we reserve judgement about whether this time these good intentions will be translated into action, and that that action will be sufficient to cure this festering abscess, which is at present a blot on the good name of the NHS."

The main recommendations made by the *Independent Inquiry into the Death of David Bennett* were:

- All who work in mental health services should receive training in cultural awareness and sensitivity.
- All managers and clinical staff, however junior or senior, should receive mandatory training in all aspects of cultural competency, awareness and sensitivity. This should include training to tackle overt and covert racism and institutional racism.
- All training should be regularly updated.
- There should be ministerial acknowledgement of the presence of institutional racism in the mental health services and a commitment to eliminate it.
- There should be a national director for mental health and ethnicity similar to the appointment of other national directors, appointed by the Health Secretary to oversee the improvement of all aspects of mental health services in

relation to Black and Minority Ethnic communities.

- All mental health services should set out a written policy dealing with racist abuse, which should be disseminated to all members of staff and displayed prominently in all public areas under their control. This policy should be strictly monitored and a written record kept of all incidents in breach of the policy. If any racist abuse takes place by anyone, including patients in a mental health setting, it should be addressed forthwith and appropriate sanctions applied.
- Every care programme approach should have a mandatory requirement to include appropriate details of each patient's ethnic origin and cultural needs.
- The workforce in mental health services should be ethnically diverse. Where appropriate, active steps should be taken to recruit, retain and promote Black and Minority Ethnic staff.
- Under no circumstances should any patient be restrained in a prone position for a longer period than three minutes.
- A national system of training in restraint and control should be established as soon as possible and at any rate, within twelve months of the publication of this report.
- The Department of Health should collate and publish annually, statistics on the deaths of all psychiatric inpatients, which should include ethnicity.

Crisis in the Community

- All medical staff and registered nurses working in the mental health services should have mandatory first aid training, including cardio-pulmonary resuscitation.
- Records should be kept of all psychiatric units' use of control and restraint on patients. The Department of Health should audit the use of control and restraint.
- There is an urgent need for a wide and informed debate on strategies for care and management of patients suffering from schizophrenia who do not appear to be responding positively to medication and we recommend that the Department of Health monitor this debate in order to ensure that such strategies are translated into action at the earliest possible moment.
- All medical staff in mental health services should have training in the assessment of people from the Black and Minority Ethnic communities, with special reference to the effects of racism upon their mental well being.
- All patients in the mental health services should be entitled to an independent NHS opinion from a second doctor of their choice, in order to review their diagnosis and/or care plan. If a patient, by reason of mental incapacity, is unable to make an informed decision, their family should be entitled to make it for them.
- The question of detention in and treatment of patients in secure accommodation should be reconsidered in order to ensure that no patient

David Burke

is detained in such accommodation unless it is necessary and that the period of each detention and the treatment be kept constantly under review.

- The Department of Health should examine, with the Department of Social Security, possible modifications to state financial assistance so that patients do not leave resident hospital care in order to obtain adequate financial assistance from the state.
- All psychiatric patients and their families should be made aware that patients can apply to move from one hospital to another for good reason, which would include such matters as easier access by their family, a greater ethnic mix, or a reasoned application to be treated by other doctors. All such applications should be recorded. They should not be refused without providing the applicant and their family with written reasons.
- There is a need to review the procedures for internal inquiries by hospital trusts following the death of psychiatric patients, with emphasis on the need to provide appropriate care and support principally for the family of the deceased, but also for staff members.
- There is a need for medical personnel caring for detained patients to be made aware, through appropriate training, of the importance of not medicating patients outside the limits prescribed by law and the need for more regular and effective monitoring to support the

108

work undertaken by the Mental Health Commission in this field.

- It is vital to ensure that the findings and recommendations of this inquiry inform all relevant parties, including the developing Black and Minority Ethnic mental health strategy.

If these recommendations were implemented fully, comprehensively and seriously, there were bound to be substantial changes in the experience of mental health services by people from Black and Minority Ethnic communities, according to Professor Sashi Sashidharan. He explained, "There will be a reduction in the number of people who go into hospitals under coercive measures, there will be a reduction in the number of Black patients held in psychiatric custody, in some of the most repressive conditions within psychiatry in this country. And we will know that evidence fairly quickly because people will be talking about it. This is a unique opportunity for the department and, I daresay, one of the last opportunities in trying to put this house in order and in trying to eradicate institutional racism from within our services." The Department of Health would have us believe that nearly all of the recommendations were indeed accepted, "at least in principle". Jim Fowles explains, "*Delivering Race Equality* was published alongside the Government's response to each of the David Bennett inquiry recommendations. The work is being taken forward in various ways, either as part of DRE or in related programmes. For example, NIMHE have piloted new training modules in cultural capability for the whole mental health workforce that should be available soon. There is new guidance on dealing with aggression, and plans to develop a system of accreditation for training. The ethnicity of the mental health workforce is monitored, and is more diverse than that of the inpatient population. And the down rating of benefits during a stay in hospital has been abolished."

Many of the recommendations contained in the Bennett inquiry report also appeared in *Big, Black and Dangerous: Report of the Committee of Inquiry into the Death of Orville Blackwood and a Review of the Deaths of Two Other Afro-Caribbean Patients,* published in 1993.

Big, Black and Dangerous examined the deaths of Michael Martin, Joseph Watts and Orville Blackwood, each of whom died at Broadmoor psychiatric hospital after being placed in seclusion cells. Although concerned specifically with Broadmoor, it did recognise many issues affecting all Black users of the mental health service. Its recommendations included the following:

- To introduce training in the control of violent incidents without resorting in the first instance to physical restraint.
- To monitor patterns of diagnosis among minority ethnic groups.
- Further research into the diagnosis of schizophrenia in Afro-Caribbeans.

Crisis in the Community

- All staff be given adequate training in all forms of resuscitation techniques appropriate to their discipline, with such training to be regularly updated.
- One Black appointee should be given particular responsibility for tackling the problem of racism in the special hospitals, to advise on the development of a programme of race awareness training and to devise an effective equal opportunities policy.
- That the hospitals develop clear procedures for advising relatives of the death of a patient and to ensure minimum distress is caused to relatives.

In the wake of the Bennett inquiry findings, Dr Stone fumed, "It's a scandal what is happening. The report *Big, Black and Dangerous* still holds. Very few of the recommendations of that report have been implemented. All the institutions in this country need to become anti-racist; racism has to be acknowledged."

Chapter Eight

"The confidence of the Black and Minority Ethnic communities, as far as mental health services are concerned, has been lost. There is widespread appreciation that it will take time and dedicated work to regain this trust and confidence, but it must be done." *The Independent Inquiry into the Death of David Bennett.*

*

Delivering Race Equality in Mental Health Care, a five-year action plan for reducing inequalities in Black and Minority Ethnic patients' access to, experience of, and outcomes from mental health services, and the Government response to the recommendations made by the inquiry into the death of David Bennett, was launched with much fanfare at the outset of 2005.

Drawing on *Inside Outside: Improving Mental Health Services for Black and Minority Ethnic Communities in England*, and *Delivering Race Equality: A Framework for Action,* it was based on three building blocks, namely:

- More appropriate and responsive services - achieved through action to develop organisations and the workforce, to improve clinical services and to improve services for specific groups, such as older people, asylum seekers and refugees and children.

Crisis in the Community

- Community engagement - delivered through healthier communities and by action to engage communities in planning services, supported by 500 new Community Development Workers.
- Better information - from improved monitoring of ethnicity, better dissemination of information and good practice and improved knowledge about effective services. This will include a new regular census of mental health patients.
- Within these building blocks were a series of specific objectives. The DRE vision was that by 2010 mental health services would be characterised by:
- Less fear of mental health services among BME communities and service users.
- Increased satisfaction with services.
- A reduction in the rate of admission of people from BME communities to psychiatric inpatient units.
- A reduction in the disproportionate rates of compulsory detention of BME service users in inpatient units.
- Fewer violent incidents that are secondary to inadequate treatment of mental illness.
- A reduction in the use of seclusion in BME groups.
- The prevention of deaths in mental health services following physical intervention.
- More BME service users reaching self-reported rates of recovery.

- A reduction in the ethnic disparities found in prison populations.
- A more balanced range of effective therapies, such as peer support services and psychotherapeutic and counselling treatments, as well as pharmacological interventions that are culturally appropriate and effective.
- A more active role for BME communities and BME service users in the training of professionals, in the development of mental health policy, and in the planning and provision of services.
- A workforce and organisation capable of delivering appropriate and responsible mental health services to BME communities.
- Two years into the action plan and the 500 Community Development Workers' posts, which were supposed to be in place by the end of 2006, were not even half filled. The employment of these CDWs was earmarked as a central component in the realisation of the plan; they were envisaged as important links between local mental health services and the communities they served. Primary Care Trusts were allocated £16 million to pay for the posts; the money appears to have been diverted elsewhere to patch up ailing NHS services.

The resignation of Professor Lord Kamlesh Patel – who immediately called for a national inquiry into

Crisis in the Community

discrimination within mental health - was another body blow; his exit provoked angry reaction from certain activists. Dr Richard Stone, a panel member on the David Bennett Inquiry, was sorry that such a senior figure couldn't get anything changed, but scoffed at the idea that he should lead a national inquiry, reasoning that it should be, "Someone who has a good track record of delivery".

Dr Joanna Bennett, a mental health expert and sister of David Bennett, dismissed the very idea of a national inquiry. "It suggests he is looking for an explanation for the discrimination within mental health services, but this has been clearly laid out in the *Independent Inquiry into the Death of David Bennett*, *Breaking the Circles of Fear* and *Inside Outside*."

Alicia Spence slammed DRE as, "A toothless bulldog which hasn't been able to deliver the agenda in terms of Community Development Workers". To hear that the programme lead was leaving was not good news. "It's probably because he knows the whole thing is not working, but it has created lucrative salaries for a lot of people," she said. There was further criticism from Professor Suman Fernando of the National BME Mental Health Network. He suggested that those who have led DRE, "Should stay put and not jump ship after getting credit and honours for starting this programme. If Lord Patel really wants to make a difference, he ought to take responsibility for what has gone wrong with DRE. His jumping ship is just not cricket". Lee Jasper slammed DRE as, "A complete disaster", a view shared by Professor Sashi Sashidharan. "Lord Patel's departure confirms what has been known for some time – that the Government's strategy regarding ethnicity and mental health has been a disaster. Apart from the rhetoric about DRE, the Department of Health has so far failed to show any real commitment to challenge ethnic inequalities in our mental health services," he commented.

*

Professor David Sallah, the national director of DRE, kept me waiting in reception at Wolverhampton University for more than 30 minutes. Shortly after introducing herself, his PA left my fate to her colleague who, every few moments, appeared at the door to offer profuse and embarrassed apologies. He was still on the phone. She would remind him of his appointment. Had I travelled far? Would I like some coffee? He shouldn't be much longer. When eventually I was ushered into Professor Sallah's office, his body language was cautious, guarded – as though I was there to elicit a confession. And for which crime would he assume guilt? For being another in the seemingly endless chorus line of Stepford-like spokespeople on behalf of the Government? For paying lip service in delivering the kind of race equality most African Caribbeans felt was absent from mental health services? So, how did he reconcile being a member of the David Bennett Inquiry panel, which recommended to the Government that mental health services were institutionally racist, with being national director of DRE, established by the same Government which rejected the aforementioned recommendation? "The Government didn't say yes or no to the recommendation of institutional racism – they said it was unhelpful." Unhelpful? To whom? Those institutional racists administering the services, or those African Caribbeans unfortunate enough to find themselves at the rough end of said services? "As far as I'm concerned there's work to be done and it's important to do it, whether the work that has to be done is defined as institutional racism or not. I recognise that it's important for some people, but my priority is to make sure that high levels of inequality are corrected." Inequality, whatever the context in which it is practiced, emanates from prejudice, unwitting or not. Did he himself agree with the recommendation that mental health services were institutionally racist? "You have to define it. It's a hugely contentious term. It would be useful if people actually defined it. It came from the Macpherson Report. Used in the context of David Bennett, the processes that were applied to David's care were disadvantageous. Hence that term. But I can't move on from that place where we have evidence to say that everything else that is happening in mental health is because of institutional racism. If the same definition is applied, I would need a lot more information to support that particular term."

David Burke

How about decades of evidence presented by both African Caribbean service users and mental health professionals? "When it comes to people from minority communities there is disparity in terms of access. In terms of their experience of services there are some differences as well. The actual outcomes of the interventions they have in mental health services are also of real concern."
An interesting if judicious usage of words – "inequality", "disadvantageous", "disparity" – straight out of the New Labour manual of verbosity. If Professor Sallah was uncomfortable with the charge of institutional racism, to what then would he attribute the problems faced by African Caribbeans when it came to access to and experience and outcomes of mental health services? "The DRE programme was set up to have a real programme to deal with those issues. One thing we're not able to say is that we can explain what's happening. We can't explain it. What we know and what is confirmed by the (*Count Me In*) census is that the figures are far too high for minority communities. There hasn't been a conclusive explanation as to why this is happening. We're trying to see, in time, if this really is the case." This defence of unawareness was again deployed when Professor Sallah was asked about the prevalence of poor mental health among African Caribbeans. "It could be to do with their experiences, the quality of housing, it could be to do with poverty – it could be a whole set of issues. I don't know. There's a claim that maybe the African Caribbean Black person experiences

mental health differently than anyone else. There's no real evidence. Another argument is that services are institutionally racist and that's why their experience of mental health is poor. You can't just say it's because mental health is institutionally racist; nor can you say the Black person is madder than anybody else."

The trouble with Professor Sallah is his proclivity for vacillation. Vacillators aren't renowned for delivering anything – which hardly qualifies him as the man to deliver racial equality within mental health. There has to be the will to drive the agenda forward, to consistently challenge the Government's commitment to eradicating the inequities in mental health, to ensure DRE is not just another initiative designed to create the illusion that something is being done. Fundamentally this is about gaining the trust of African Caribbean service users in a system that has failed them; it's about introducing whatever measures are necessary within that system to afford these service users – and indeed all service users – the best possible care. Remember, we are talking about some of the most vulnerable individuals in society; they need to know that the people entrusted with alleviating their suffering are doing so without bias.

Professor Sallah inherited leadership of DRE from Professor Lord Patel, whose resignation as national director of the Department of Health's BME programme was prompted by what he regarded as a lack of real progress. He explains, "When I joined the House of Lords it became a difficult situation. Mental health legislation was coming, there was going to be some conflict of interest. In a sense I was inside the department. The future was obviously going to be challenging some of the things I didn't like about what the department was doing. And it felt uncomfortable to me, as part of the legislate of this country, to be working in the department on this particular programme."

Since his departure, Lord Patel has warned of "a kind of apartheid" in the system, emphasising the urgency in addressing the claim of institutional racism. "We're going to have a situation where we'll have segregation. We'll have those that live on the margins of society feeling more hopelessness than they do now. A kind of apartheid will happen in the next ten to twenty years. It is going to get worse. We have to deal with it very strongly." He wants a public inquiry into why BME service users are so grossly over-represented within mental health services. As a member of the House of Lords he can lobby the Government to initiate such an inquiry without being compromised as figurehead of the DRE programme. "There is an argument not to have the inquiry because we've had 25 years of careful research. I don't believe we have. I believe we've had ad-hoc pieces of work that have looked at particular episodes of psychosis or geographical cities where there have been problems. We don't

Crisis in the Community

have a consistent answer to it. What I want a public inquiry to do is for a group of experts in their own field - not the usual suspects, maybe an economist even – to look at everything that's going on, to look at the literature, to look at the evidence, talk to some of these young people, talk to service users, talk to families, look at the international evidence and ask some searching questions. It's not about apportioning blame but actually asking, what do we do about it? We might never find the answer. But if we don't we have a real problem. I doubt this is to do with mental health. I think this is to do with society. If we can't begin to attempt to ask that question, we have a real problem. We're not going to deal with the whole issue of cohesion and terrorism. We're never going to deal with all the issues around shootings. We're never going to touch the mental health stuff because we don't know where the problem lies. I've got an open mind. I think a lot of the problem lies from primary school to adolescence. But I have a completely open mind about it. I'm prepared to look at everything and find some solutions to it. And I can't believe any Government wouldn't want to do that. I will continue to push this because it has to happen. In the end I'll go and seek private funds for it, but I don't think that's the right way to do it. Government should want to know why we have this situation. And until we know that there will be bits of DRE that always have a gap. DRE will work structurally fine. But there will always be gaps in understanding what's happening. I do feel gutted about the idea of not leading this. But to me, leading is about leading. I want the power to make changes. I want people to listen when I say these changes need to happen. And I want the resources to do it. It guts me to see hundreds of people doing some super work. It's a lot of the young people who are leading this now. A lot of the older people like me, some of them are too cynical. I think there's a lot of anger. I could easily fall into that. Something always stops you, whether it's money or politics. A lot of anger has built up over the years, but that's not going to move us on."

Professor Sallah seemed to concur with Lord Patel's call for a public inquiry – or did he? Navigate your way through the fog and arrive at your own interpretation. "What will we have if we have an investigation? We will be taking information from people telling us things that are wrong based on very little information they have. My view is that a real study should be commissioned of why it's happening, to find out in a rigorous way why the case is the way it is. It would have to be external to DRE. DRE is more to do with changing the situation as it is now. It's the first time there is a programme to deal with this."

And change was happening, according to Professor Sallah at least. There was more community engagement and better information being provided to mental health services, enabling them to plan comprehensively the effect of their interventions. "And we're making sure that the way of obtaining information about what happens in mental health services is refined to include stronger representation for minority communities."

Many delegates at the second annual DRE conference in Coventry were more wary of what had been achieved. Hari Sewell, director of social care partnerships and focused implementation sites at Camden and Islington Mental Health Trust in London, responding to the second set of *Count Me In* statistics, which virtually remained static from the previous year, asked, "What are we going to do with these statistics? Are we going to keep saying nothing has changed, all the way to 2011?"

Angela Linton-Abulu, project co-ordinator of the Black Women's Mental Health Project, was considerably more scathing. She described DRE as, "One of the worst toothless things I've seen in a long time, a scandal from day one. There's no commitment to dealing with people that are excluded and over-represented in terms of resources." And Professor Sallah's response to any criticism of DRE? "People have a view and I'm quite welcome of that view – it keeps me on my toes. All I ask people is that if they are going to criticise, they use the evidence. What we so-called leaders of the minority communities say has a real impact outside that circle of how people view mental health services. At the end of it we have to have treatment for mental health problems in every community. If people say mental health services are racist or discriminatory, all that will happen is people won't use the services. More people who are ill won't have access to services early. There are consequences to what they're saying."

Crisis in the Community

Chapter Nine

Delivering Race Equality is just another initiative. An important one, admittedly, given that it was drafted in response to the *Independent Inquiry into the Death of David Bennett*, itself a watershed in the African Caribbean experience of mental health. But it will not fix a problem that is merely a tributary of a bigger societal problem: the racial stereotyping that continues to inhibit the successful integration of African Caribbeans into the so-called mother country.

He may no longer be directly involved with the programme, but Professor Lord Kamlesh Patel continues to champion it – with one proviso. "I think DRE is still the best thing I've seen anywhere in Europe or the rest of the world in terms of a systematic response to dealing with a major inequality and a scandal in the health system. But it is not an answer to all things. It's a panacea. What we have at the moment is anything that happens in the mental health world that's associated with race, it's up to the DRE to solve it. DRE is not going to solve everything. We can't set it up to fail in that respect. It's doing a super job, but there are other things that need to happen alongside it."

Maxie Hayles, chair of the Birmingham Racial Attacks Monitoring Unit, one of his many personas during four decades as an activist, feels there is a lack of will to deliver race equality in society, let alone mental health, among local and central Government. "Take the 1976 Race Relations Act," he says. "Campaigners such as myself considered it toothless for what it was. It took the murder of Stephen Lawrence to get an inquiry, whereby Judge William Macpherson made representations which led to the strengthening of the act in 2001. But having done that, what keeps me awake at night is the fact that it's not really been implemented as it should. Some local authorities haven't even considered addressing impact assessment. Unless you do impact assessment you cannot see the gaps in service delivery. In terms of service delivery, they have to have the will – the political will – and that will help the situation. But we don't have that. We have piecemeal initiatives. There are no sanctions. Heads should roll. The act recommends that local authorities make provision to address gaps in service delivery. It's not been implemented. The Commission for Racial Equality are culprits in this. They were supposed to be the ones taking this forward. But now it's got even worse. The CRE has disbanded. A group of us actually buried it down in London. We had a mock coffin - we drove around the city with this coffin and buried it. We read a eulogy over it as well! There is no safeguard for Black people in terms of obtaining justice the way the Commission for Racial Equality and Human Rights (the CRE's replacement) is set up. Yet they're the ones who are supposed to take the initiative of the strengthening of the 2001 act and take that forward. We need an alternative."

Hayles believes there has been too much "pussyfooting" around the issue of race, and that this will not change until those in authority make "painful decisions" and invest some meaning in punitive sanctions. "For instance, how many times is someone going to call someone a Black bastard and say they didn't mean it, that they were drunk or it was just a one-off? They kick the Black man's arse and then they say they're sorry, that they unwittingly did it. And then they do it again. Then there are no sanctions. We need zero tolerance. If you really want to address it, you have to clamp down on it. After all, Britain colonised two-thirds of Africa. This country should be a beacon, leading by example. They made more money from slavery than any other country. The British Government could come clean and redeem themselves in order for us to move forward in a civilised manner. The Atlantic slave trade, which is still impacting on us today, has to be remembered rather than cast aside."

The African Caribbean community can move forward themselves by taking ownership of their problems, according to Hayles. We know racism exists. We're not going to harp on it. But in order to move forward, you have to look where you're coming from. You can't quarrel with history because it's gone, but you have to remember it, you learn from it. You have to ensure that it doesn't happen again. The teaching of Black history is to benefit everyone. White people need to understand where Black people are coming from. Every Government that takes power in this country insist that children learn about 1066 and the history of that. And unless you can balance it out by teaching the history of Africa, you have not got a level playing field."

*

Dr Roi Ankhkara Kwabena describes himself as a cultural anthropologist, but really he is so much more. Of Trinidadian origin, he has worked all over Europe, in Latin-America, Africa and the Caribbean for the past thirty eight years on a variety of issues, including the therapeutic harvesting of memories by elders and young people, anti-racism, community cohesion, social inclusion and refining the heritages of indigenous peoples. In the mid-nineties he served as a senator in the parliament of his home country. A poet of some renown, he was Birmingham's Poet Laureate in 2001. Throughout his extensive travels he has never encountered any one group of people as troubled as African Caribbeans. "They're the most traumatised people I've met on the planet. When one looks at the situation in Africa, particularly in Sudan, where they have famine, problems of war, problems of so-called terror, Islamisation, genocide, the people are not as much traumatised as African Caribbeans here in Britain. It's down to the absence of family life, the absence of community, the absence of support systems that are so necessary for communities such as ours. If you don't have a demarcation line between a child, a teenager, an adult and an elder, and you have a problem with the traumatised situation facing people with their memories and the whole thing about disappointment, it causes problems in the family, community, and, therefore, society. Remember, the people who came to these parts during World War I, during World War II and after World War II, to the mother country, are sorely disappointed. The image had been implanted in our consciousness that here was paved with gold, and it's not. And the other thing about the mother country, as the coloniser it implanted Christianity on the mindset of those people, and they really hold fast to that faith. They came here expecting to be embraced in the church, and they were spat out. Basic tenets of religion, like the commemoration of the crucifixion of Jesus, which people believe in, that whole thing about Easter and Lent, these weren't practiced here as they were in the Caribbean. This is an industrialised society that doesn't place the kind of value on these kinds of traditions." Societies in Africa have retained traditional systems despite colonisation. For Dr Kwabena, it's all about identity – that word again. "People who have been deprived of their memory and transplanted to the Caribbean, who have had to make a new world for themselves and have survived successfully to the extent that they have contributed towards the redevelopment of this place as professionals, weren't accepted.

They were made to clean hospital floors, clean train stations and be spat upon and be lumped alongside Irish and dogs, and not given equal opportunity in the mother country. Even people who have made great strides in terms of being prominent – Lord Learie Constantine (cricket legend, political activist and Britain's first Black peer), CLR James (journalist and social theorist), people like that – they faced racism here. And it was a shock for them. Even though they got knighthoods, out on the street they faced racism. Lord Constantine wrote a book on the colour bar – his family was thrown out of a hotel in London. He told them he was a knight, but they didn't want to hear that. My strength is culture. And I believe that humanity is developed from community level and family level – a woman, man, child, family, community and nation. If these things are totally disrespected and they're not considered equal when it comes to certain parts of the planet, there will be consequences."

So why is there no perceived community among African Caribbeans here? Why are African Caribbean families so fractured? "The divide and rule tactic has been successfully used and there are a lot of wounds that have not healed. One of those wounds is a post-traumatic slave situation. It's something that needs to be addressed, without reparations, without an apology. Even in the Caribbean at the moment we have a fall-out in terms of crime. But that has a lot to do with a kind of neo-colonisation or neo-imperialism. If you go

Crisis in the Community

back to the Caribbean from England, the first thing the community will say is that you're mad. Because many people who have returned to the Caribbean, they come back dishevelled, they come back traumatized, they come back unable to fit back into the society there. A lot of people who are born in this country of Jamaican parentage who regard themselves as Caribbean, when they go back there they're not Caribbean."

Dr Kwabena is a practitioner of cultural literacy, a concept based on the premise of mutual understanding of and respect for cultural difference. It is also about self-respect. "If I don't respect myself, how can I have respect for you? I'm not going to come to you with a chip on my shoulder, or come to you on wounded knees, like a victim. There's a world of history in which Black people played an important role, in which all oppressed people played an important role. Cultural literacy crosses all barriers of race, class and gender. It's about empowering people to understand that they mean something, that they are important, they are valid, that they have made a contribution. "And when I say 'they', I'm talking about your ancestors – our grandmothers, our grandfathers, our great grandparents – who did something so that we could be here today. If it wasn't for their struggle, we wouldn't be here. So, we give credit where credit is due. We make a level playing field. If we recognise our sameness, if we can recognise that we have a responsibility to the ones to come and the ones that are here, the younger ones, then we could start the ball rolling. It begins with me. And I'm seeing ripples. It's a way to begin to heal the wound. And the fall-out of that wound is mental illness."

African Caribbeans, according to Dr Kwabena, see themselves as victims; and this is compounded by their experience in British society. "Everywhere you look among African Caribbeans here there's a lack of self-respect, an inferiority complex - bleaching cream, wigs of all sorts, fashion that looks intolerable. A complete lack of identity - an identity crisis. How we are going to repair that? That's serious work to do. And then the state talks about multi-heritage, ethnic, BME communities – they're always appropriating these terms and names for people. African people in this country from the Caribbean, looking to the holy land of Ethiopia, many of them get a chance to return and they pack the baked beans and chips in their bag!"

The identity crisis Dr Kwabena talks about, as well as national, is also familial, he believes. "There was a problem with the African Caribbean family unit in terms of the way it was done. Men came here from the Caribbean and then they sent for their wives, or they didn't send for their wives and then they got into marriage here. And then you had the instance of children being allowed to be reared in the Caribbean and then sent for to meet brothers and sisters they didn't know. Plus, I have talked to young people about their childhood and

Crisis in the Community

the way they've been treated in the educational system, and the problems they were confronted with in the class and that they were disbelieved by their parents, because their parents had the mindset of our teachers."

It is this familial factor to which Dr Kwabena alludes as a causal factor in the disproportionately high levels of mental illness among African Caribbeans. But even more destructive is post-modernism. "Poor mental health among the African Caribbean community is the result of an industrialised society that don't see themselves as post-modern. That's a form of madness too. I think Europe is currently in a state of crisis. It doesn't know whether it's coming or going, and then it comes up with this new term, post-modernism. "When I was a child, they told me I'd be living on the moon. When I added up my age I thought, I'm going to be too old boy, because man had just landed on the moon. But when I look back at my community, people are still carrying water on their heads. Where's the modernity there? And they're drilling for oil and gas, right next door to where they're living. It's all about a society of consumers. Everybody wants to consume at all costs necessary. And consumerism is a contributory factor to mental health."

Dr Kwabena is appalled to think that people are sectioned under the Mental Health Act on the basis of race in this post-modern age. "I am appalled too by the lack of cultural literacy of the people who sit in positions of power within the system to make the decisions. Let us say a person has a mental illness. They go to the hospital and say they have a problem. They're sent to the next person to tell their whole long story. Then they're sent to the next person to tell their whole long story. And then they put up a cultural illiteracy barrier, where people draw assumptions. The people drawing these assumptions are poor, they are oppressed, they are White; they got no power but they got a job. And they're not doing their job properly. And they're drawing assumptions and making decisions that can affect a human being's life. It's the way society has been constructed. Racism is based on fear. It's all about power. I put on some plays developing cultural activities to empower my people. Amongst them are some very talented people. One day I met one of my actresses walking the road, trembling. She's been sectioned. She's been pumped up with injections. Why? She's an enthusiastic person. Enthusiasm is not respected in this country. In another case, I heard of a young man who had been sectioned because he washed his rice seven times. Now washing the rice is a tradition in my country. Who came to that decision to section that guy?"

*

Maxie Hayles has a couple of hypothetical examples which serve to emphasise the detrimental effects of misreading indicators of cultural difference, not to mention the absurdity of entrusting decisions regarding someone's mental health to non-mental health professionals. Section 136 of the Mental Health Act, incidentally, concerns "mentally disordered persons found in public places" and states: "If a constable finds in a place to which the public have access a person who appears to him to be suffering from mental disorder and to be in immediate need of care or control, the constable may, if he thinks it necessary to do so in the interests of that person or for the protection of other persons, remove that person to a place of safety." Hayles explains, "Take, for instance, on a Sunday morning, a person may have been to the blues the night before and they may stand up and they start snapping their fingers. They've got the boogie in their bones and they're feeling good. The police can come and arrest you under Section 136 of the Mental Health Act and take you to a police station. There's a cultural thing in the West Indies where people get messages, dreams, to go and warn the world that God is coming and you must repent. That person could be taken to a place and considered mentally ill. It's wrong diagnosis usually. They don't know anything about African Caribbean culture, yet they're the ones who are assessing and diagnosing. They have a misconception of Black people, stereotypes backed up by an unjust justice system that we have in this country, which reinforces that stereotype, criminalising Black people. It's a failure to come to terms with their racism. For years, anyone with any sense of humanity has been fighting and trying to put some sense to the misdiagnosis of African Caribbeans. It seems to me there's a Government conspiracy to keep Black people, a certain amount of Black people, incarcerated with a label. You have to think it's a political conspiracy at times. What else would stop people from seeing the reality of injustice? What's going on there? They don't want to admit to it. They're not meaningful. They pay lip service. They've lost the will to improve the lives of Black people in this country."

Hayles, a redoubtable campaigner for the African Caribbean community, doesn't see much cause for optimism either. That a figure of his unyielding faith in the ability to change wrong into right appears to be losing hope for the future, is a stark reflection of how betrayed African Caribbeans feel by the guardians of society. "I am usually optimistic. But when it comes to race and White supremacy, I'm a bit sceptical. The jury's out. We have to empower our young people to think strategically to overcome that. This is a psychological thing. We have a constant psychological battle to prove on a daily basis that we're even human beings - forward ever, backward never. But many Black people pretend and deny; all they want is their belly full. But what we're doing is towards posterity, to make life easier for generations to come and make them more acceptable. If not, it's just going to perpetuate itself over generations.   We need to stop that cycle of ill will."

Chapter Ten

The word 'racism' runs through this book like the noxious effluent from a sewer; it's impossible to ignore. Most of those I spoke to had no compunction about acknowledging it almost as a fact of their existence; nor were they in any doubt that it has had a corrosive impact on the African Caribbean psyche. The fact that those damaged by the hostility that underpins racism, whether overt or not, are then funnelled through a mental health system, in which it is institutionalised, is a shameful indictment of a society that perceives itself as being among the most civilised on the planet. The slave trade may have been abolished two hundred years ago, and slavery itself may now have gone underground, but the contemptible ideology that galvanised it continues to fester in the sub-conscious of its descendants; of course, in these enlightened times its manifestation is absolved by its unwittingness.

Dr Joy DeGruy Leary, an assistant professor at Portland State University in the United States, espouses the theory of post-traumatic slave syndrome, a kind of inter-generational trauma based on post-traumatic stress disorder. The systematic dehumanisation of African slaves was the initial trauma, she claims; and generations of their descendants have borne the scars ever since. Some of the criteria used to diagnose post-traumatic stress disorder – the sufferers of which are rape victims, war veterans, victims of natural

Crisis in the Community

disasters and severe accidents – are strikingly similar to behaviours exhibited by African Americans. These include diminished interest or participation in significant activities, a feeling of detachment or estrangement from others, irritability or outbursts of anger.

In America, Dr Leary charges, an acute social denial of both historical and present-day racism has taken on pathological dimensions; the country, she says, is, "Sick with the issue of race". Dr Leary explains, "The root of this denial for the dominant culture is fear, and fear mutates into all kinds of things: psychological projection, distorted and sensationalised representations in the media, and the manipulation of science to justify the legal rights and treatment of people. That's why it's become so hard to unravel. Unfortunately, many European Americans have a very hard time even hearing a person of colour express their experiences. The prevailing psychological mechanism is the idea that because I've not experienced it, so it cannot be happening for you. Truly, how can anyone tell me what I have and have not experienced? This is a very paternalistic manifestation of White supremacy, the idea that African Americans and other people of colour can be told, with great authority, what their ancestors' lives were like and even what their own, present-day lives are like. The result for those on the receiving end of this kind of distortion is an aspect of post-traumatic slave syndrome. People begin to doubt themselves, their experiences and their worth in society because they have been so invalidated their whole lives, in so many ways."

Multi-generational trauma is not a new concept. Dr Leary refers to the Holocaust and how it is acceptable for Jews to make sure it is never forgotten; she compares this to how Blacks are told to let go of slavery. "The reason that there is such a level of discomfort between Whites and Blacks is because we are a reminder to them of their barbarism. One society that is responsible for some of the most gruesome crimes against humanity in history is the United States of America. While the powers that be are happy to talk about other people's crimes, they seem reluctant to confront their own."

American journalist John Head, who spent twenty years living with untreated depression and now works to increase awareness of the condition within the African American population, is another who subscribes to notion of post-traumatic slave syndrome, believing that the brutality of slavery and the unending humiliations of segregation have exacted a terrible toll on the mental health of African Americans.

Dr Alvin Poussaint, a professor of psychiatry at Harvard Medical School, directed a psychiatry programme in low-income housing developments in Boston, Massachusetts in 1967. Black people often refused him entry to their apartments; they feared and mistrusted a medical system that had been used to oppress them, especially with the use of involuntary hospitalisation. At the same time, Dr Poussaint recalls, many clinic workers were afraid of Black men, so gave them the most severe diagnoses "just to get them out the door". He continues, "Blacks are over diagnosed for psychosis and paranoid schizophrenia, but under diagnosed for depression. Racism is interwoven into everything."

The African American experience is not so very different from the African Caribbean experience here in Britain. And Head's assertion that America is "paying a high price for neglecting Black mental health" sounds ominously familiar. As Dr Poussaint clarifies, "People today who lack feelings of self-worth devalue their own lives, but they also devalue the lives of other Black people. At least 85 percent of Black crime is committed against other Blacks. Homicidality in Black youth results from devaluation, hopelessness, isolation. The problem is, we don't consider anger a mental health issue, but there is a lot of chronic anger out there".

*

There are advocates of the post-traumatic slave syndrome on this side of the Atlantic, among them Dr Richard Stone. He ascribes many of the problems encountered by African Caribbeans to slavery. "I come from a Jewish background. It's very interesting that we hugged the Holocaust very much to ourselves for 50 years. In the last ten years Holocaust survivors began to realise they must talk before they die out. These people had great secrets in their families. When there are secrets in a family, they can be immensely emotionally damaging. We're beginning to realise how damaging this is when people don't talk about it. These secrets damage people's relationships and their health. In slavery, the men were separated from the women. So when you talk about Black men in this country not standing by their offspring, not standing by their women to bring up their children, I have a feeling a lot of that is rooted in slavery. Plus, the fact that when people came to this country, the man was sent over first. Ten or fifteen years later the mother would come with the children. When I talk to Caribbean friends of mine about what their grandmothers told them about what their grandmothers had told them, you're going back six generations; these were often women and men in slavery. You realise the traumatic effect of what had happened with the men – the men were never involved, and many of the women were demeaned and raped by their slave masters. And the traumatic effects have gone down through generations."

Dr Stone belongs to the Black Jewish Forum. About ten years ago, during the Jewish holiday of Passover, the group hosted a special Passover feast for its African Caribbean members. The attendees included Lee Jasper, senior policy

Crisis in the Community

advisor on equalities for the Greater London Authority, who had just returned from a trip to Ghana. Dr Stone remembers, "I asked what he thought about all of this. He said that the amazing thing was the ritual of the washing of the hands. You have a ritual where you wash the hands without a prayer, and later on you wash the hands with a prayer. I asked him why that was so important to him. He said, "Don't you understand - our families were uprooted; they were people of great ritual and we've lost all our rituals". All the ancient rituals of Black people have been wiped out, except in Africa, although even there many have been wiped out due to colonialism."

Dr Roi Kwabena is another who feels that post-traumatic slave syndrome has never received appropriate remediation. He says, "In the absence of cultural literacy, descendants of chattel slavery had had inaccurate psychological assessments as mental health service users. Further, these foreign theories are all Eurocentric and do not address the cultural sensitivities of service users in so-called mother countries, independent states and colonies. Clinicians still use Freudian and other theories that have no pertinence to the diverse experience of non-Europeans. The false concept of superiority and maintained position of non-committal responsibility for the introduction of that unjust system and its subsequent systems – for example, imperialism and capitalism – contributes directly to the psychosis that is endemic to communities still marginalised. After the so-called abolition of that dastardly trade in human cargo, nothing was done to address the resulting trauma which was genetically passed on to the descendants of the sufferers. Instead, other systems were introduced, such as apartheid and social segregation. Even in my own lifetime lynching was still carried out in America. Authoritative practitioners all agree that one does not have to live through an experience to be traumatised by it. So, in the absence of resolution, deviant attitudes and behaviours resulting from trauma can be passed on through generations sub-consciously. Self-hate, dysfunctional families and interpersonal relationships, and anti-social behaviour are all consequences of post-traumatic slave syndrome."

Professor Kwame McKenzie, a senior lecturer in transcultural psychiatry at University College London, isn't convinced by the post-traumatic slave syndrome argument, but certainly feels it needs to be researched. Professor McKenzie identifies Prime Minister Gordon Brown as the one politician who could initiate such research and, in so doing, move away from the controversy surrounding reparations which dogged the last months of the Blair administration. "Reparations is a cul-de-sac argument that people have," he says. "I'm a researcher and a psychiatrist, so before we talk about reparations, we need to know what there is to repair and we need to have some idea of what we need to be doing to repair it. What should happen is we start off with money going

Crisis in the Community

into a fund which looks at the long term effects of slavery. Once we start understanding that, then we can have a proper debate. Let's be sensible about this. It would have to be a big project. If someone was a big thinking politician – and Gordon Brown is not long after taking over as Prime Minister – trying to think of how we move this forward, this is the sort of thing he should be doing. Why are there so many Black people in prison? Why is there so much gun crime? Why are Black people disproportionately represented in mental health? Some people are saying it's inherited trauma. That might or might not be the case. We don't seem to have a huge number of answers as to how to sort this problem out. It costs 50 grand to keep someone in prison for one year. It costs 150 grand to keep someone in a psychiatric unit for one year. And there are a lot of Black people in psychiatric care units and in prison. Maybe we should be pumping money into proper research to find out where this is all coming from."

There has, as Professor McKenzie points out, been a lot of research on genetic memory and its far-reaching effects. "Say, for instance, you are 12-24 weeks in-utero and your mother suffers trauma. You, as a child, have to be prepared to deal with that trauma. Her high levels of adrenalin and other hormones get transferred through the placenta. That changes the reactivity of your serotonin and your own adrenalin functions in your brain as a child, increasing your reactivity. That's one of the ways you move stress from one generation to another. Once you've got this high reactivity, the question is whether you pass it onto your children – there's quite a lot of evidence to show that you do unless your social environment significantly changes. The initial problem is that trauma that happens to your mother completely changes your genetic expression. That's what's called an echo-genetic effect as opposed to the hardwired big gene change. We know there are echo-genetic effects in wider society; we know there are social changes that cause long term problems. So this sort of theory, which seems ridiculous, becomes something that might be worth having a look into. It's not an excuse for people deciding they are going to leave their kids, or for people losing their temper, or for drug taking – it's not an excuse for anything. But it is a possible explanation. And generally it's useful to know where things might be coming from in order to produce short term, medium term and long term solutions."

Studies conducted after the Second World War found that babies in-utero at the time of the Nazi invasion of Holland who were in the third trimester, had an increased chance of developing schizophrenia. "We know that people who have been a victim of racism have smaller babies. We know that something is going on. I'm not saying there is a Post-Traumatic Slave Syndrome. All I'm saying is if there is a major holocaust that has specifically affected one part of the population, then it is going to be important to see if there are long term scars that we need to know about and sort out."

Another sceptic is Professor Suman Fernando. His reservations concern the medicalisation of slavery, the implication being that Black people are "patients of sorts". The medicalisation of a social experience is one of Professor Fernando's principal objections to post-traumatic stress disorder itself. "I think I would rather see White people as suffering from delusions of grandeur, or superiority, because of slavery. Admitted to that, apologising and paying compensation for it could help. In fact, one could see slavery as a sin or a grave injustice done to Black people, leaving White people with a burden that may amount to illness. Expiation is a way out of sinfulness. I do not think it an advantage to see Black people as damaged, sick people. It is White society that is sick."

David Burke

Chapter Eleven

Black Mental Health UK was established in 2006 to raise awareness and address the stigma associated with mental illness. The group's objective is to reduce the inequalities in the treatment and care of African Caribbeans, and furnish them with information on how they can influence the strategic development, policy design and implementation of services. Briefly, Black Mental Health UK wants to enable the African Caribbean community to improve the Black service user experience, and lower their over-representation at "the coercive end of psychiatric care". Its many supporters comprise the Black Police Association, the Black Londoners Forum, The Afiya Trust, The African Caribbean Evangelical Alliance, The National Assembly Against Racism, The 1990 Trust, The Mental Health Alliance and The African Caribbean Mental Health Commission; from outside of Britain there is further support from Black Brits USA and Facilitators for a Better Jamaica.

Fronting Black Mental Health UK is Matilda Macattram, a woman of formidable faith in the ability to change the mental health experience for African Caribbean service users. Macattram won't contemplate the possibility of failure in the pursuit of what she regards as a human rights issue. Ultimately she wants to see a mental health ministry birthed out of the Black Mental Health UK campaign; she will not be appeased by tokenistic measures, not when the blood of David Bennett is "screaming from the ground". She says, "He represents so many people we don't know about. People are dying when we're at peace. The NHS is a world class service. People in America look at the NHS and think, wow. In America, people die because they don't have medical care. That doesn't happen here – it's not supposed to. People might slag off this country, but the standards are outstanding, and yet this is allowed to happen? It's not an isolated incident. This pernicious, horrible thing is just eroding the good work of good people. There are some good people with good hearts. Not everyone's a racist, not everyone's evil, not everyone has power trips. There are some really, really good people, but this stuff is eroding their good work. I see people doing incredible work. But there are just pockets of good practice, where there's no stigma, there's no demonisation, there's no over-medication, no misdiagnosis, no condemning the families, no police sirens coming along and restraining people - there's none of that coercive, evil stuff that comes with mental health care. There's just speaking to the family, finding out what the problem is, supporting them through the process, seeing people recover."

On the whole, according to Macattram, the African Caribbean community is choosing not to engage with mental health services. "Why should you engage in something that's going to make you come out looking like a vegetable, if you don't come out in a body bag?" Consequently, many suffer in silence when they need treatment because of the very nature of the treatment meted out to them in the mental health system. This silence, Macattram claims, is another way of keeping people in bondage. "People say that African Caribbeans are culturally different. How different can some young boy be who was born and bred say in Battersea, grew up in South London, was educated in either the public or private education system in this country, goes to university, leaves, and yet because of the colour of his skin he's now culturally different? How culturally different can you be? They're not different, they're British. The system as it is set up is racist because it will discriminate against people in a certain way. Mental health services do not function in isolation. You have pathways into care. You can go in voluntarily, which I wouldn't recommend anyone does. The stories I've heard... If somebody you know has a breakdown, I would so not recommend it from what I've heard. And then you can go via the police, the criminal justice system. If you're in court and you're perceived to have diminished responsibility, you can then be referred to a mental health hospital rather than to prison. For African Caribbeans you are 50% more likely to be referred to mental health services through the criminal justice system. We know sentences and ethnicity. You can go via the police route. The 1990 Trust produced a report for the Metropolitan Police Association which shows that African Caribbeans

Crisis in the Community

are six times more likely to be searched than a White person, even though it doesn't lead to an arrest. We're looking at the pathways to care. The BBC documentary, *The Secret Policeman*, showed quite clearly that there are new recruits who think Stephen Lawrence deserved what he got. The mindset has not changed that much. Given the mindset of the people who are the gatekeepers, it shouldn't really come as too much of a surprise that the treatment of the most vulnerable – these people are the most vulnerable in our society – is being done by someone who has a perception of them that's negative. And then they don't have any recourse to somebody who, let's say, had the education and the financial resources - all the stuff you need to protect yourself. People can do what they want. What's happened to us as a community is we've found ourselves en masse in the worst place you can be if you're living in Britain today. That's not why we're on these shores."

But using Martin Luther King and Nelson Mandela as inspirational touchstones, she is adamant that African Caribbeans shall indeed overcome. "It's not just an ideal; it's the objective that will be attained. This country is based on statutes that are all to do with righteousness, truth and justice – it's enshrined in law. We're going to get what we want. Like with lots of things you want, you have to go through stuff, don't you? Things like truth, righteousness, justice; it's not only about believing them but knowing that they will out eventually. We have enough bodies. The deaths in police custody, the over-medication, the sexual violence... People on the outside have to do something. Because do you know what? Right now, somebody's going to be sectioned and they're not going to be mad; they might have had something to smoke, or they might not be mad at all, and they're going to be in a situation in a hospital. There's one person I know, he went to the GP. You know young people do certain things? Well, this guy was playing on his Nintendo, so he's starting to fry - I'm sure there's a medical term for it, when somebody's spaced out and can't sleep. He's not feeling well, so he goes to his 'baby mother' - he's got a relationship with this woman who has his child but they're not co-habiting. He's not registered with a GP. So she says, "Go and see my doctor". So he goes down to see his partner's doctor. You've got to remember, he's fine. He's a bit spaced out. People say rubbish when they're lucid and it's a normal day. So he gets this letter, he goes down to this place and some people come up to see him, they're wearing white coats. This is an African Caribbean guy in his early twenties at the time. He said these two Black guys came in, two guys who worked there, and they said, "You're staying". He says, "No, I'm not". The next thing he remembers is he woke up, he was naked and there were pyjamas beside him. He was in the system for about five years. And right now someone else is going to find themselves in that situation. We're in powerful positions whether we realise it or not. We can use that to give a voice to the voiceless."

Among those in the "powerful positions" to which Macattram refers is the media, which can wield particular influence in a free society – if it chooses so to do. Again she uses the campaign for civil rights in the United States to demonstrate her point. "The land of the free, the home of the brave, America. People were like, "'Let's go there and make money". Then people found out that Black people couldn't sit at the same counter as White people. They didn't realise about all the lynching – there's all this stuff they didn't know about. And then, because the media exposed the dirt, there was pressure from outside as well as from inside. That made it change." But surely the idea of crusading media intent on spearheading the righteous fight against iniquity is a throwback to a bygone era, a time before corporate manipulation of media organisations dictated content? Hasn't truth been sacrificed on the altar of greed? "Everything's evolving. We're evolving, the world's evolving and we're learning and we're growing. And they will all come out and fulfil their destiny." Such an opinion requires a huge investment of faith – faith eroded, for example, by the media's collusive role in the invasion of Iraq. "Faith I have! Not only do I have faith but I have evidence of people who've done it. And they're the examples I will follow," asserts Macattram.

Chapter Twelve

For a period of ten years between 1989 and 1999, Gilroy Brown was a rarity in British education – an African Caribbean headteacher. Brown, who decided to become a teacher to change the system from within, forcing it to recognise the Black presence in and contribution to society, not only substantially raised standards at Foundry Road Primary School in Birmingham, but he also employed a minority ethnic staff at all levels. Yet his pioneering efforts, rather than act as a spur to the educational establishment to involve more African Caribbeans at the highest level in its schools, seem to stand as an exceptional example of what could be achieved in this regard. The 2007 Wanless Report, as outlined earlier, painted a disturbing picture of underperforming Black pupils who were routinely punished more harshly and praised less, and were three times more likely than their White counterparts to be expelled permanently. "The impact this has on poor mental health among African Caribbeans goes very deep," Brown says. "What you have at the end of the day are young people with a huge sense of failure and a sense of hopelessness. The hype is that school is not cool. Many young Black men see school as playing by the White man's rules, and so they reject it, but they reject it at their own cost. Many young people leave school feeling despondent and disillusioned because they haven't achieved anything, they have no prospect for the future. They see their White peers, by and

Crisis in the Community

large, succeeding. As long as the gatekeepers, when it comes to people who are not like them, don't have the interests of Black pupils at heart, these pupils are always going to be marginalised and kept out. The present gatekeepers now are going to have to give people like me space and opportunity. And they ain't going to do that, because an opportunity to me is a threat to them."

Brown's not sure if it's overt racism or plain ignorance on the part of what he terms "the host society"; but from the perspective of African Caribbeans, there is suspicion of its erstwhile oppressor. "History does affect your psyche, the way you behave. History of oppression, where you have to fight your rights, your right to be a human being, from the day dot; where the enemy that's held you captive, tried to destroy you and been your constant nightmare for generations, where the stories that your forebears pass down to you, telling you to watch out for the enemy, that they're still there to destroy you. You'll fight for survival, you'll fight against all the odds, you'll fight no matter what it costs, for your dignity and your humanity. And central to all of that, an integral part of it, is your sanity. If that's constantly under attack, you don't have the luxury of living like a normal human being. For me, I think the biggest challenge for many Black people in this country is trying to stay sane. In one sense the easiest thing is to let go and go insane. For most oppressed people, it's the same kind of thing. You go insane and you fall right into the trap that's been waiting for you. It's of no concern to the powers that be. Many people came over to this country from the Caribbean expecting the streets to be paved with gold. Some quickly adapted and adjusted, because you've got to survive. Others never got over it. Some became disheartened and crazy - they passed that onto their kids also. I'm not making excuses. Look at the media. The only way in which a Black person can make it is for them to act the way the White man wants him to act. It was the minstrel back in the twenties and thirties, now it's the gangster rapper. Where's the difference? You've still got to appeal to the host society. You can't be ordinary and straight. I was a headteacher for ten years – the only Black male headteacher of a Birmingham primary school. The people who've got the power don't want to see people like me because I don't fit the stereotype. Sadly, many of our young people subscribe to the ghetto gangster hoody thing. Individuals are not allowed to be themselves and are being forced to live out a stereotype. That's the only way they can survive. If you are essentially not like that – if you're a gentle, sensitive, basically law-abiding person – then you have a problem, because you're playing up to an image."

There, once again, is the conflict of identity that so many African Caribbeans I met while researching this book spoke about as being an inescapable fact of the community's disproportionately high rates of mental illness – that, and the legacy of the

Crisis in the Community

slave trade. "For a long time I thought we were making excuses when we talked about the impact of slavery," Brown admits. "But when you think slavery was only abolished over a hundred years ago, in the course of history and evolution, that's like yesterday. It's bound to have an impact on subsequent generations, and it will have for the next several hundred years if there isn't a fundamental change in the way society is run. If there's anything out there to reinforce the fact that you're still not free, to remind you that you're not worth more than the dirt on the ground, that legacy is going to have greater resonance."

Brown believes the onus is on people like him, African Caribbeans who have "made it" to some extent, to be more vocal in furthering the community's aspirations; for only when African Caribbeans feel that they genuinely are stakeholders in society, that they can accomplish their objectives without prejudice, will their overall psyche improve. To this end, Brown, along with former graphic designer Guy Woolery, established the KWESI Mentoring Project in the early nineties. They engaged 50 Black men from all walks of life, the youngest being 24, the oldest about 70, who could mentor and work with Black pupils in schools. This is part of what Brown sees as the twin strategy of revolution and persuasion. "The days of the riot are dead. Even during the sixties – and I used to follow the fight for equality in the United States during the sixties - as much as it was great to see African Americans fighting for their rights, there was a downside as well. Some inner city parts of the States now still have to be repaired.   The Government were punishing people, in a sense – if we dared to tear their buildings down, they would show us. I think there has to be protest. Protests and riots are two different things. Protest on a number of levels. People like me; we are able to speak out where the masses won't be able to. We have the ear of the gatekeepers - they have to respect us because we've qualified to be there. You've got to be a representative for African Caribbeans and speak out in the right circles. The problem is that too many people are too concerned about not rocking the boat. I do feel there are creative ways of protesting. Strategically, for example, we've got the Race Relations Amendment Act, which the community has not used to its advantage. I think we should test it out – I don't think we test it out enough. I also think the Black churches could have a lot more to do. If you look at the situation in the States, the Black churches in the States played a very instrumental role in the fight for civil rights. The Black church in South Africa, in the fight against apartheid, did the same. That's the missing element in the African Caribbean fight for freedom, equality, justice and respect here in Britain. More needs to be done. The Black churches need to form an alliance with other secular Black organisations. At the moment they're working in isolation."

*

Crisis in the Community

Claire Felix is the former national leader of race equality at mental health charity Rethink, which works to help everyone affected by severe mental illness to recover a better quality of life. She has a somewhat fatalistic view of the African Caribbean male experience of mental health, believing a whole generation has been lost because of the authorities' failure to confront not just racism within institutions, but racism within British society. "We have research going back twenty years. We're going to have to rebuild generations. I think we have lost a generation of African Caribbean males. They don't have family, they don't have wives. They've become disenfranchised from their families as a result of their illness. These are guys who've spent many years in the system. They've been permanently damaged. They are languishing out there in our community. But race is something that it's not politically correct to be talking about - the level of disadvantage that exists amongst particular groups," she says.

When it comes to mental health, African Caribbeans don't consider the system to be caring or sensitive to their needs, according to Felix. "There's a fear of statutory services. There's a fear of authority in general. African Caribbeans are least likely to go for help early. They wait. With African Caribbean families it's often the mother or a family member who recognises that this person obviously needs outside help, or when they become a danger to themselves at home.

The first port of call is often the police. By the time they do gain access to mental health services they're already at the severe end of the illness. So they experience difficulties in terms of accessing services. When they're in there they don't build up trust with professionals, trusting relationships. The first opportunity they get to disengage from the services, they do, on discharge. They have expressed dissatisfaction with services. They experience poorer outcomes in every area of mental health. They are detained longer. And the diagnosis frequently changes. They're more likely to be deemed more dangerous. The other thing is that they experience difficulties in recovery. Once they leave hospital and get back out into society it's difficult to get back into society, to get back into being included. It's almost a double whammy."

Bleak though Felix's analysis of the African Caribbean relationship with mental health services, unlike Gilroy Brown she does feel that there is a sense of solidarity among African Caribbean community groups and a real desire to be at the forefront of change. "African Caribbeans are more likely to come from broken homes. We know that there's a huge percentage raised by lone parents. Parents who have had their children young and spent a lot of time at work didn't spend a lot of time with them as children. Long hours, parents often away. When they go to school, particularly African Caribbean men, they end up underachieving, which means that their life chances are reduced. As a community they feel disenfranchised. However, we also have to look at the resilience in African Caribbean families. They are strong. Communities are coming together now as a group and saying they want to see change. That's not something they've done in the past. They do have views and those views need to be considered by policy makers."

She is cautious in recognising that *Delivering Race Equality* may be a step in the right direction. But those entrusted with administering the programme have to, "Be more responsive and look at the experiences and hear the narratives of people who use services". And, of course, this first entails accepting there is a problem with institutional racism, something which, as outlined already in these pages, the Government considers unhelpful. "With DRE, you're problem solving – and institutional racism is the problem. Acknowledge that it's there and then look at the structures. More work could be done in terms of early intervention by working with African Caribbeans from a younger age. Youth clubs, where you teach young people mediation skills and emotional intelligence - those things are important. It needs to be done with communities. We'd need to re-establish the concept of youth clubs in the first place. You'd need to work with whole communities and talk to them about what they need, talk to the youth themselves, form youth councils. Give them a voice in those services. Give them control of those services.

David Burke

Mainstream services need to look at how they're delivering services – far more outreach needs to be done, far more engagement with those communities. I'm looking at the school curriculum and embedding mental health in it – understand mental health, the signs, the symptoms, the causes of it. And Black history is important too. It allows African Caribbeans to have some pride, to look at people who achieved before them. It is possible to attain, to achieve and be a successful individual. We don't have enough of that. We don't celebrate our achievements. There are some people doing fantastic work in the community. We don't hear about them, but they are there – the unofficial social workers on the ground. The more difficult it is for African Caribbean males to break those barriers they have in life, the more they will increase because they will turn to other ways to manage their emotions. There needs to be an acknowledgement that it's wrong and we want to change things – we're serious about wanting to change things."

Crisis in the Community

Chapter Thirteen

The tragic story of Michael Powell (known as Mikey) is, in many ways, the story of how not only the mental health system has failed African Caribbeans, but the story of how Britain has failed African Caribbeans, of how White perception of Black is principally governed by stereotypes. And of the genuine fear among African Caribbeans of mental health services. As long as this prejudice on the part of the White community, and paranoia on the part of the Black community, remains the case, African Caribbeans, together with most other ethnic groups, will feel dislocated from British society.

In summary, Mikey, a cousin of poet and novelist Benjamin Zephaniah, died at the age of 38 while in the custody of police in Handsworth, Birmingham. The father of three young children, he had never been in trouble with the authorities and was a well respected member of his local community. He was, though, susceptible to bouts of depression, one of which occurred on the night he died, 7 September 2003. "It's something that's going to be with my family for the rest of our lives. It's something we're going to have to live through," says his sister, Sieta Lambrias.

*

Mikey Powell was more like a dad than a brother to his younger siblings growing up in Lozells,

Birmingham. Instinctively protective, he always made sure they were aware of the dangers that existed on streets that, years later in 2005, gained national notoriety for the race riots between African Caribbean and Asian youths. Even back when the Powell youngsters were growing up, Lozells had a reputation. It is a sad reflection on human nature that areas, often on the basis of superficial evidence pieced together through rumour, and moral panic initiated by sensational media coverage, tend to become blighted. As a consequence, good people's lives are made more difficult as they struggle to carve out an existence. But the Powells, according to Sieta, never had any problems in Lozells. "Mikey was always well respected in the community. As a teenager everyone knew Mikey Dread - they called him that because of his locks. He was never in gangs or posses. He was well known, well liked and just got on with it," she recalls. "As he got older and had his own children, he just carried on the same way. He pretty much lived for his three boys. As a teenager, and going into his twenties, he didn't have a job. Then the minute his first son came along, that was it – he was out to work, off to support his family. He became really responsible. He said, "Now that I've got children, I've got to provide for them". And he did. He started working – labouring-type work mostly. He knew it wasn't the greatest type of work to do, but he knew that nobody would look after his children but him. He stopped going out. He would rather stay in with his children. His partner would go out with us and

Crisis in the Community

he would babysit. That was year in, year out –
working, taking the boys to school, babysitting at
the weekends. He was at home a lot of the time.
Looked after his family, looked after our mum.
Mikey was mum's favourite - and she would admit
it. Mikey would do all sorts of odd jobs for his
sisters – decorating, he'd take them shopping. He
did an awful lot of running around for all the family
as well as his own kids."

They were a close-knit family, spending birthdays
and Christmas together, debating together, with
Mikey invariably making himself heard above the
din. The image Sieta conveys is one of a man
who was content to occupy the roles of surrogate
dad, good son, big brother, protector and provider.
Whatever mental turmoil he was going through, he
kept it well hid from his family. "To my knowledge,
Mikey didn't have a battle with depression. If he
was going through some battle, then being
protective he wouldn't have wanted anyone to
know what was eating him or if he had any
problems. Until that night, in that particular year, I
didn't realise that he was having any problems at
all. My sister and my mum were there with him
and for three or four days he was feeling quite low
and something was troubling him. He'd gone to
the doctors, but I wasn't aware of that until the
fatal night."

Mikey had "three or four episodes of mental
breakdown" over a ten-year period. "The first time
he said there were voices bothering him. He went

through 48 hours of being troubled by something in his head. He never actually got to the bottom of it. We took him to the Priory in Edgbaston. I wasn't going to send him to (psychiatric hospitals) All Saints or to Highcroft. I wasn't having it. You take a Black man into a place like that and that's it. They'll inject him with all sorts and then he'll come out even worse. I was brought up in Lozells. I've seen it. I witnessed on my road a family that had four sons similar in age to us. I'll never forget one of the boys, he used to hang out with my sister when they were teenagers – they used to go scrumping and have play fights and all sorts of fun. And he was as cool as a cucumber, this guy. Next thing you know he ended up in Winson Green Prison for burglary. This was over twenty years ago. About a year later he came out and he was walking along the street like a zombie. I thought, oh my God, what have they done to him? He was always quite vocal. The story was that in Winson Green if you talked too much, if you defended yourself, they'd inject you to calm you down. Black guys were being injected to calm them down, and whatever drug they gave them calmed them right down to cabbages. And I witnessed that back then as a teenager. I could see a man who, as a boy used to laugh and joke with us, get mixed up into the wrong crowd, do some robberies, he's gone inside, he won't keep his mouth shut and apparently he's been injected. It was awful to see. He was as low as anyone could be a completely different person. So when Mikey had his first episode there was no way I was going to take him to All Saints or Highcroft to be injected. He needed help. Obviously he had something wrong in his head. They were not going to inject him with drugs and ask questions later, so he ended up like a cabbage. There was no way I wanted that. We took him to the Priory. They asked us if he smoked weed, we said he did. They couldn't see too much more wrong with him. They weren't sure. We said he was seeing things and hearing voices. We told them we didn't want him injected, just wanted him given some medicine-type thing to calm him down. Four days later he was out and that was it."

Following this, Mikey experienced two more episodes, neither of which Sieta was around to witness. "I was living away at the time, but the story I got was that he'd climbed onto the roof and started taking his clothes off. The fire engine came and got him down. They told him to go home. Two days later he was alright. He had episodes once every four years or something. The episode on the night he died would have been the fourth one. Two or three days before, he was talking about going to the doctors. He didn't feel well, he had stomach ache. The doctor gave him some Gaviscon. It was that kind of thing. We don't know what was troubling him. Unfortunately, Mikey's not here, so we don't know if it was going to be a full-on breakdown or if it was another episode."

At the time of his death Mikey was staying with his mother. He and his girlfriend were having relationship difficulties. Sieta believes this may have been a contributory factory in his worsening psychological state. "He was suffering at the time. That night he's come home and sat with mum and my sister Jude. He seemed really calm. Mum and Jude went to bed. He was watching TV. Then they heard a smash. When they came back down Mikey had smashed the front window of the house, smashed the coffee table. He climbed through the window of the house and then started to smash his own car window. It's gone eleven at night. Mum's in her seventies, Jude's seven months pregnant. Mum's worried - there's nobody around except mum and my sister. As a pensioner you'd think, I'll phone the police and get some help. That's exactly what she did. She called the police, told them she needed some help that her son had lost his head, that he'd smashed the window, smashed his car and that he was wandering up the road. That was the nature of the call – it was an appeal for help."

By the time the police arrived Mikey, having walked up the road from his mother's house, was on his way back again. His brother-in-law, Junior, having been summoned by Jude, was also on the scene. "Junior knew that Mikey wasn't well. He turned up to make sure everything's alright. Luckily for us that Junior did turn up at that time, because he witnessed absolutely everything the police did. There were two of them in a car.

Crisis in the Community

Mikey was walking back down the road, his hand was bleeding. The police car drives past him, slows down as it drives past. Mikey hits the back of the car with his hand. Whether it's to tell them to stop... who knows? They've driven down a bit. There was a mini-roundabout where my mum lives. They've gone round that, turned round and come back up. Mikey is now outside my mother's house. And Junior's talking to him, asking him what's going on. Mikey was walking towards the police car in the middle of the road. Junior says Mikey's hands were at his side, the police said his hands were behind his back. Mikey's walking in the middle of the road towards the police car and they drive at him and knock him over. They knocked him over the bonnet. They said in court that they'd knocked him over because they thought he had a gun. So he hit the car, went over the bonnet, fell down at the side. They reversed, he got back up again. He then staggered towards Junior. They then called out. Junior's holding him, and then they cross the road. They got out of the car. Bearing in mind they thought he had a gun, they actually came out of their car and walked towards him. They ran towards him, beat him with batons, CS gassed him, pinned him on the floor. Several other officers turned up in a van. Witnesses say there were between four and six on him. The police admitted there were at least four of them on him. So now he's face down, being suppressed, after being CS gassed, beaten with a truncheon and knocked over, on top of having some mental problems."

Junior was powerless to intervene, having been CS gassed as well. "There was so much CS gas sprayed that two of the officers had to sit down on the curb. If they were overcome with CS gas, and Junior's eyes were watering with CS gas, what do you think Mikey was suffering? "People were telling them to get an ambulance. They pinned him down. They handcuffed him. The family was stressing that he needed help, that he was mentally unwell and needed to be taken to the hospital. They were pleading with the police not to harm him. Mum, who'd called for help, was witnessing all this right outside her front door. Then after a very long time he was put in the back of the van. It had seats but the officers, rather than put him in a seat, laid him across the floor. They put him in the back of the van and drove to Thornhill Road Police Station. He was handcuffed. They said he was fidgeting, there was movement, he was jerking – so they knew he was alive. He could have been gasping for his last breath, we don't know that. We never found out in court what happened in the van because the Crown Prosecution Service didn't push it in court, because they had no evidence. So we don't know what went on in the van. He got to the station and he was carried out by five officers. In my opinion, based on the CCTV footage I saw, he was already dead. They said they did CPR on him. They were basically saying he was unconscious, not dead.

Crisis in the Community

Why didn't they take him to a hospital? That's what he needed. The next thing we hear, an officer turned up and said Mikey was dead. So two hours after being called for help, a fit, healthy, 38-year-old, who had mental problems that needed looking into, was dead. We will never know what he was going through, and that's what angers me the most. Mikey needed treatment and what he got was abused by the police."

*

Ten police officers faced a range of charges following Mikey's death. These included dangerous driving, assault and misconduct in a public office. All ten were acquitted at Leicester Crown Court in August 2006, the majority of charges having been dismissed on the direction of the judge; he disallowed crucial prosecution evidence of the transcript from the custody CCTV audio, deeming it unreliable because of its poor quality.

In April 2007, the Independent Police Complaints Commission confirmed that none of the officers involved would face disciplinary charges, a further blow to the Powell family's pursuit of justice for Mikey.

John Crawley, IPCC Commissioner for the West Midlands, said he was aware, "Of the gravity of the matters at stake, the suffering of Michael's family and their dignified endurance and unfailing courtesy", adding that their sense of loss was, "As acute today as the day Michael died". Fine words indeed, but ultimately hollow as far as the Powells were concerned – and made even more so when Crawley spoke of the police officers' trauma.

As for the reasoning behind his decision not to initiate disciplinary proceedings, he explained, "The evidence for any misconduct hearing would be essentially the same as that considered at the trial, and I have examined the findings and outcome of the trial very carefully indeed. I am satisfied that in this particular case, and given the weaknesses in evidence against the officers that the rigour of the criminal process exposed, their acquittals should suffice in terms of the formal accountability expected from these police officers."

*

The Powell family still don't know the official cause of Mikey's death. There has been no inquest. "Nearly four years later and we're trying to get the coroner to sort out a date for an inquest," says Sieta. "Four pathologists handed in reports. One couldn't decide what killed Mikey. Another said it might be a blood thing. Another one said they didn't know but they didn't think the officers did any harm. And a fourth, the family pathologist, said he believed it was more than likely positional asphyxia. If it was positional asphyxia that would have happened when he was put into the van."

Crisis in the Community

Mikey's death has politicised what was once an apolitical family. Yes, the Powells are getting on with life, as they must, but life now incorporates The Friends of Mikey Powell Campaign for Justice, an organisation dedicated to ensuring that the truth will out eventually. "As well as Mikey's campaign, we campaign for a group against deaths in police custody, and Black people and mental health. Black people have got issues around mental health and how they're targeted. If there's a Black man or a Black woman shouting too loudly, it's a case of, 'We've got another mad one here'."

Mikey's mother, Claris, and eldest son, Rio, have been particularly affected by his death. Rio, thirteen at the time, vowed then that if justice was not done, he'd complete his schooling, study law and reopen the case. For Claris, the heartache of losing her oldest boy, and in circumstances in which she inadvertently played a part, won't ease. "My mum will never get over it. The fact that Mikey was her favourite child; coupled with the fact that she made the call... she'll just go to her grave with that. That's the worst ever thing that could have been put on my mother. She placed her faith and truth in the police, the people who are here to serve the community, to protect and serve the community. It would have been better if it were a stranger. But the police... Mum is of a generation, what else does she know? For me, the first generation of West Indians born here, I

173

would have put him in the car and taken him to hospital myself."

Crisis in the Community

Chapter Fourteen

A 1999 inquiry into social exclusion and mental health problems by Mind found that the arts, "Can play a catalytic role in promotion social inclusion, both by virtue of the participatory processes involved and the products created". Sound Minds, based in the London borough of Wandsworth, is a social enterprise which applies that principle to improving the lives of people under the care of community mental health teams. Its services include sessions in music technology, production and recording, DJ-ing, visual arts, movie making and editing, drama and poetry, as well as other arts projects. "We are reclaiming the arts from therapists, releasing the talents and voices of our members," according to a spokesperson for the organisation.

Sound Minds began in 1992 on the site of Springfield Hospital in Tooting when inpatients established a music group and gave performances in the library. A year later, community occupational therapist Libby Notley was attending a non-mental health community networking forum on a Battersea estate, when she met local Methodist minister Peter Sharrocks. He told her of a music studio in the basement of his church. At this time the studio had some commercial use, and was also frequented by youth offenders and a drugs rehabilitation project. Notley and another occupational therapist, Kieron Corrigan, had a number of people in their caseloads with musical ability who were unemployed and not interested in either training or existing mental health facilities, among them a former guitarist with reggae star Dennis Brown's band. It was decided to rent the basement studio once a week for two hours. This proved so popular there was a waiting list of people wanting to take part. Consequently, a second group was established in 1994, this one staffed by occupational therapist Paul Brewer and Devon Marston, a mental health service user, actor, guitarist, bassist and drummer.

Twin disasters struck shortly afterwards when the basement was flooded, thus diminishing broader community and commercial use of the premises, and there was an armed robbery in which £10,000 worth of equipment was stolen. The venue's volunteer manager and other staff, both traumatised and disillusioned, resigned their positions, leaving the mental health groups as the sole remaining tenants. At this stage the waiting lists stood at 27 people, two thirds of which were from ethnic minorities; 100% of those either attending or on the waiting lists had a medical diagnosis of a psychotic illness, and between them had an average of 2.5 hospital admissions each. The minister of Battersea Methodist Mission put forward the money acquired from the Church Urban Fund and the Methodist Mission Alongside the Poor – a total of £12,500 – to found Sound Minds. The local health authority also contributed funds. The studio was re-equipped and a full-time studio assistant employed.

Crisis in the Community

More than a decade on, Sound Minds – a registered charity and a company limited by guarantee, the majority of whose staff and directors are service users – is funded by Wandsworth Primary Care Trust, the Big Lottery Fund, Comic Relief and Wandsworth Adult and Community Learning; these monies are supplemented by performances, workshops, conference appearances, and art and graphic sales.

*

Devon Marston was seven years old when he arrived in Britain from Jamaica. Several months after joining his family here, he learned that his grandmother – who had raised him until that point – had passed away back in the Caribbean. Her passing would have a devastating effect on Devon's mental health, though not until he had reached his twenties. By then he was homeless, jobless, drinking heavily and a habitual marijuana smoker. "I left home when I had a big row with my parents. They didn't approve of where I was going - I was starting to grow my hair and smoking a lot, and I was big into my religion," Devon recalls. He cut a shambolic figure on the streets of South London. "I was grieving for my grandmother. It was delayed shock. She was such a big part of my life."

It was his brother who persuaded him to make peace with his parents, inviting him round to the family home for dinner one evening. While there, his mother called the local GP round to examine him. A second doctor was also summoned, this one accompanied by two policemen. Devon became alarmed upon learning that they were taking him to hospital – Springfield psychiatric unit.

After being admitted Devon was medicated heavily. He slept until it was dark. "When I woke up I didn't know where I was. So I went to ask a nurse if I could go home. She became frightened and pressed a buzzer. All of a sudden these four white men came into the ward. They held me down and injected me." Devon reckons he was unconscious for some four days, during which time he claims he "nearly died". "When I came to I felt like I wasn't Black anymore. My spirit had left me. They were turning me into a White man. I was always a conscious Black man. But now my mind didn't feel the same. And physically I was in a lot of pain. I was crawling around the floors on all fours, slobbering all the time... my trousers were falling down."

Devon stayed at Springfield under section for six months, his positive response to medication culminating in his eventual release. There have been relapses in the past twenty five years or so, though these have occurred when he has stopped taking his medication of his own volition, "Whenever I thought I could manage without it" – something he realises will never be possible.

Crisis in the Community

While Devon agrees that the racism he experienced as an African Caribbean in seventies' Britain – he was labelled a "Black bastard" by a teacher when he turned up late for a school trip in primary school, and frequently had to endure "gollywog" taunts from classmates - probably contributed to his mental illness, he prefers to cite his lack of identity. "I learned all about Queen Victoria and stuff like that in school, but I learned nothing about my Black heritage. I only found out about my own Black culture at home. That's the same for not just all African Caribbeans but Asians as well."

Mental health services are, in Devon's opinion, stained by an absence of cultural awareness; again he is disinclined to use the word racism. "Of course, racism is part of it, but mostly it's about mental health services not understanding where Black people are coming from. And the most important thing all service users need is care – we need people to listen to us."

These days there are more young African Caribbeans, especially men, being referred to mental health services than ever before – a marked contrast to when Devon was first sectioned. "Back then it was mostly older people. But nowadays service users are getting younger and younger. I think a lot of them are in the system because they smoke too much and drink too much." Sound Minds, more than the intervention of his family all those years ago, proved to be Devon's redemption. "It has helped me to sort myself out. I picked myself up and started again with Sound Minds. It's an example of the kind of thing that can be done to help Black service users."

*

"It's the only job I've ever been for that said you had to have a mental illness to apply," says Coral Hines of her position as house manager at Sound Minds. "They know that if you have mental illness, it's never going to go away. You never know when you're going to end up in hospital." This was certainly true in Coral's case; her first, frightening spell in hospital having been in Israel – where she'd gone to work and stay in a Kibbutz - at the age of nineteen when "out of the blue" she became ill. "I started hallucinating, singing... I was elated, I was on air. I was so high – it was wonderful. Everybody thought I'd been taking drugs. They carted me off to a psychiatric hospital. I was put in the secure unit. I didn't know what was going on. I was strapped to the bed, injected straight away and just left. Then another injection came around... That's how it was for ages. You were strapped to the bed, face down; you'd have an overall and it opened at the back. They just used to come along, lift it up and give you an injection. I didn't know what I was being given. I didn't have a clue what was going on."

Crisis in the Community

Coral had had no previous history of mental illness. "I didn't even know what it was. I didn't know it existed." Eventually, after about nine months, she was accompanied back to Britain by someone from the Kibbutz. Rather than find treatment for her condition on returning home, Coral actually found herself homeless. "My foster parents were away on holiday and the children's home that I had been in said I couldn't go back there to live because, the age I was, I should never have left. But they did let me stay there for a while. My foster parents came back but they couldn't really cope with my behaviour. It was just off-key. I was eating them out of house and home. Everything they had to eat I was eating it. I would even eat my foster parents' dinner that was left in the oven. The children's home was just a little way away, so I would go up there and eat them out of house and home as well. The medication was making me do that. I had no help whatsoever when I came back to Britain. I didn't know what to do. It was foreign to me. I didn't know where to turn. After that, I came to live with my mum, and she lived in London. I was there for a little while, then I had another episode and ended up in Springfield Hospital. I was there for a year, came out and had no support. I had a social worker for about three weeks, and she said, "Oh, you're alright now", and that was it. When I had my son in 1986 I got really ill, so I ended up in there again. The treatment in Springfield was awful, diabolical. Absolutely diabolical. I was put in rooms that were no bigger than a toilet, without any toilet facilities, on my own. They just locked the door and they went. You just literally had a mattress in there. They said I was bi-polar, which is manic depressive. At one point I was pumped with Valium, straight into my vein. I couldn't move from where I was. I couldn't smoke a cigarette, I couldn't do anything. I know that maybe my behaviour was aggressive or flamboyant, sometimes OTT. I might have needed some help in terms of restraint. But they just literally went over the top."

Coral took part in group therapy sessions for a while. "We used to talk in groups. But I was so ill I found it no help to me whatsoever. My thinking was not that realistic, so I couldn't really relate to what they were saying or doing. I was just bored. I needed to be doing something, engaging in an activity or something. Maybe a sport or a bit of music or play. But that wasn't offered. At one time they put me in a room and they had all these soft toys. I found that I could play in there. They didn't need to medicate me because I'd use up all my energy in that room and bring myself down. But they don't use it now."

On her last admission over a year ago – her previous one having been eight years before – Coral noticed changes. "Things were still a bit off, but on the whole they treated me so well. You could tell they genuinely cared about people. They would do things they weren't supposed to do for you. Some of it was still rough. The staff

Crisis in the Community

would help you all the way. That was really, really good. I really was happy with that service. Things do change, but they go so slowly. But they're still really quick to give Black people heavy doses of medication, where they wouldn't necessarily give that to a White counterpart. I'm a big girl and I've had four big men restraining me. When I tell them they're hurting me, they're putting on the pressure more. And I've had that not just from White nurses either - one of my worst experiences was from an African nurse. I think it's the fear that causes damage. Where somebody might be just getting irate, White people put it down to something that it isn't. Misconception."

Coral may never be free of her mental illness, yet nor is she captive to it. This she attributes to the therapeutic approach at Sound Minds. It was her salvation. "I hit rock bottom. I had just lost my job as a home help with Wandsworth council because they found out I had mental health problems. I was at home looking at the four walls. I had no friends. I had just moved to London, I didn't know anybody. I told my key worker I couldn't take much more of it. He suggested joining Sound Minds. They accepted my application. I used to go there once a week and sing in the reggae band, Mission Impossible. Then we started getting a few gigs. We changed the band's name to Channel One. Then I got a job as the cleaner there. Then I left to have my daughter. After that I got really ill and had to spend another spell in hospital. I came out and went back to Sound

Minds. The job as a cleaner had gone. They made another post of house manager and I got the job. I've been doing that for thirteen years. Now the band is well established. We've got loads of gigs." Coral doesn't know what she'd do without Sound Minds, doesn't know how she'd cope with her illness. "It's brought me from rock bottom right to the top. It's been an open door. Everybody just gets on with everybody. I couldn't pay for the service I get at Sound Minds. It's totally supportive if you want it to be. It is what you want it to be."

Crisis in the Community

Chapter Fifteen

Professor Kwame McKenzie's research background prevents him from becoming too emotive about the African Caribbean experience of mental health. He deals in data – the kind of data culled from carefully constructed investigation – and considered conclusions. There is a cerebral detachment in how he conveys what he has learned. Many of the subjects who participated in this book were animated when discussing the subject. Matilda Macattram was completely confident in what she knew about how mental health services were damaging African Caribbeans, yet her faith in the inexorable march towards a resolution – rather like the faith displayed by the American civil rights activists she admires – was steadfast. Maxie Hayles, jaded by decades of inertia on the part of the authorities, wasn't so jaded that he couldn't still get riled. And Dr Richard Stone was heartbroken by what he heard at the David Bennett inquiry, and heartbroken further by how little has been achieved since the inquiry panel published its findings.

Professor McKenzie is different – he's not given to anger, sorrow or the kind of conviction that's rooted in the notion of the truth ultimately emerging triumphant. He is an unflappable character, yet such is the weight of his arguments, he is the most convincing of interviewees. Which is why, when he declares that mental health

David Burke

services will improve for Black and Minority Ethnic service users in general, and African Caribbeans in particular, heads nod in agreement. This declaration, like others he makes, comes from a pragmatic place. Anyway, more anon; for now, he articulates the case for poor health among African Caribbeans. "There are two different things going on. There are common mental disorders such as anxiety and depression. And there are compulsive disorders. These make up the most of what you see as mental distress. And then there are very severe mental illnesses, which are psychotic illnesses such as schizophrenia. When you look at the rates of depression and anxiety, it's very difficult to find higher rates in people of Caribbean origin in the UK. If you look at the rates of suicide, these figures are very difficult to find because we don't have ethnic groups on our death certificates – we only have country of birth. But from all the indications there are not high rates of suicide in people of African and Caribbean origin in the UK. However, when you look at psychosis, you do find high incidence rates – high rates of new illness. However, when you look at community surveys and you try and find how many people are in the community with the illness and are ill at any one time, you don't find higher rates. Or if they are higher rates, they're not much higher – they're double as opposed to five to nine times. The incidence rate is five to nine times, but the prevalence rate – the number of people actually in the community with higher rates – is about twice. So there's something going on,

Crisis in the Community

which seems to be that there are certain specific social stresses that lead to people of Caribbean origin having more incident illness, but then also being more likely to get to fully recover. That's why you get the high incidence but the marginally raised prevalence. There are loads of factors. Studies show that if you are a migrant you have an increased risk of developing psychosis of about two to three times. So all migrant groups have increased rates. If you are a Black migrant to a White country, that rate goes from two to three to between four and five. So that starts making you think that it's not just migration itself, but on top of it, being Black has a part to play. When looking at migration we're looking at problems of separation from family and certainly separation from your parents when you're young. Then you look at socio-economic problems. Then you look at problems to do with culture and culturation. So there are all these normal problems that you have – education, getting housing, getting into jobs, getting money, being considered bottom of the pile, and also feeling an outsider. Another risk factor for developing psychosis is living in a city. And ethnic minorities and migrants tend to live in cities. So all of those are important. On top of that, for people who are Black, there's a risk of racism. There's fairly good work which shows an association between being the victim of racism and developing psychotic symptoms. There are a number of different things going on. One is straightforward racial abuse or racial attack. About 14% of ethnic minorities claim that they've been a victim of racial abuse or assault in any one year. But on top of that – and that will increase your rate of psychosis two-fold – there is this idea of perceived cognitive racism. For instance, one study asked people whether they thought that the majority of employers would discriminate against you because you were Black or Chinese or South Asian. That was a big study of about 5,000 people in the UK. If you were the sort of person who said, 'I think they would', which is about 40% of the Black population, that increased your chances of developing psychosis, or having psychosis, by about 60%. So it's not just actually having a racist attack or racial abuse. It's ending up with the cognitive schemer which says, people discriminate against me, life if unfair, that increases your chance of developing psychosis. Of course, it could just be that all you're finding in these kinds of studies are paranoid people. There was a study in the Netherlands. They got 5,000 people. Found anybody who had a mental illness and said, "We won't follow you up". Found anybody who had a paranoid personality and said, "We won't follow you up". And then they asked people if they had been the victims of discrimination. That could be racial discrimination, sexual discrimination, sexual preference discrimination, discrimination because you're fat or discrimination because you had a disability. They could be any of these things. You're followed up for three years. The people who said they had been victims of discrimination didn't have mental illness and weren't paranoid. They were more

Crisis in the Community

likely, three years later, to develop psychotic symptoms. These are well people with no current psychiatric illness, no history of psychiatric illness, no paranoid personality. They were just asked if they were victims of discrimination. Not only that, if you had been the victim of discrimination in more than one area, you were about five times more likely to develop psychotic symptoms over the next three years. So, you can imagine how being discriminated against economically for being poor will interact with being discriminated against by your racial groups. These things interact over a period of time to produce an increased chance of developing a psychosis. Most people who develop a psychotic symptom never see a psychiatrist. Over a year's period, if you look at places like Maastricht in the Netherlands, 15% of people will have a psychotic symptom. Sometimes they're due to drugs, sometimes they're due to grief, sometimes they're due to the fact that they have some sort of illness. But most people get them and they go away. What seems to happen is if you develop a psychotic symptom, but you have a number of other problems such as socio-economic problems or other stresses, those symptoms are less likely to go away. They're more likely to stay and you're more likely to end up needing help. The amount of help you need depends on the cohesiveness of your family and your community. People of Caribbean origin in the UK do not have cohesive communities. They're poor and they don't have cohesive communities. Not only do they have risk factors for developing psychotic symptoms, a lack of cohesive community is a factor. They have a high percentage of people living alone – loads of single mothers. The lack of a social support network means those symptoms are more likely to become chronic. And, the final coup de grace, when they go to their GP, their GP is less likely to offer them any other treatment apart from direct transmission to a mental health hospital or a psychiatrist. Now, all of our studies where we're looking at the incidence of illness are based on first contact with mental health services. So when you put it altogether, there are the risk factors, the perpetuating factors that produce chronicity, and then on top of that there are the transmission factors of moving people from being in the community into the glare of psychiatry. And that is why people of African Caribbean origin are more likely to end up with a diagnosis of psychosis."

Bad enough that African Caribbeans are more vulnerable to developing mental illness in the first place, but when they access mental health services – mostly through referral rather than voluntarily – this illness is exacerbated by their experiences. Professor McKenzie blames it squarely on the lack of plurality within the system. "There are problems to start off with in terms of pathways to care. So by the time people have turned up, people don't want to be there because the mental health services have got themselves a bad name. That's why many of them go not via their GP but via the criminal justice system. And when people turn up having gone through that system, the mental health services get very worried about risk, and therefore start off with a relatively negative attitude. The services have one way of treating people. People in the Caribbean population will tell you they're under stress, they'll tell you there's racism, and they'll tell you there are loads of things out there that are causing them to be stressing out. The service will tell you they're going to give you more medication. And people say, "Well, just a second... if you can get me better education, some social support, some life planning, and try and decrease the racism, I think I'll be alright". The services say, "But we don't do that. What we do is give you medication". So you get this circular argument where people are saying, "You're not giving us what we want", and the services saying, "You're ungrateful for what we're giving you". And it goes nowhere. I think a significant problem with regards to the services is there needs to be more plurality in the services, and they need to listen to what communities want, then they wouldn't have these problems with pathways to care."

Professor McKenzie was involved with Antenna Outreach Service, a culturally specific mental health service for both African and African Caribbeans aged between sixteen and twenty five suffering from mental illness. A multi-disciplinary team comprising a consultant psychiatrist, senior psychiatric social worker, senior registrar in psychiatry, mental health nurse, occupational technician, youth worker and family support co-ordinator worked with rather than on behalf of the service users – an ideal of the kind of service Professor McKenzie would like to see available on a wider scale. "It was set up with community involvement. We surveyed the service users and asked them what they wanted. What they wanted was work, job planning, relationship help, stuff that was going to be positive around their culture, and then maybe some medication, or a doctor to see them. And once you started doing that, all of this stuff of people having difficulty engaging, you didn't see too much of it. People would come and see you because they'd dropped out of school and they thought they could get access to home tuition, which they could. But if you got home tuition you also got someone from the service coming to see you once a week. It wasn't a problem. You knew what people wanted, you provided what they wanted, they turned up, you saw them, you got early intervention and treatment. But the services are not flexible enough to meet the challenges of a multicultural society."

Not only are mental health services too rigid, but as repeated throughout this book, they are tainted by the charge of institutional racism levelled at them by the David Bennett inquiry panel. "I find it almost impossible not to agree with the Bennett inquiry's finding that mental health services are institutionally racist. If one has DRE, and DRE is an institutional framework for improving mental

Crisis in the Community

health services and we've got a lot of evidence of disparities, and we're saying the way to get rid of these disparities is by this institutional response, which is DRE, then we must have some sort of institutional racism. We're saying we have disparities, we're saying they're institutional and there's an institutional solution; as far as I can work out, that means we've got institutional racism. An example would be if you're a refugee or an asylum seeker and you don't speak English, or anyone who doesn't speak English. At the moment I have someone who's Chinese on my ward. We need to get a Mandarin interpreter. We can't have a Mandarin interpreter for four days. But he speaks no English. Is that an individual problem? Can I sort that out? No. Can the nurses sort that out? No. It's a problem with the institution, which hasn't produced a structure by which you can get a Mandarin interpreter. We can only work inside the system we're given. We can shout about it, but it is actually the system – an individual cannot sort out that problem, unless we're going to learn every language. The institutions have to sort these things out. If a person ends up on a secure psychiatric ward, and nobody is able to communicate to them while they're there, what sort of care is that? These things happen all the time. Getting hold of interpreters is a basic problem. Getting support for refugees and asylum seekers is a basic problem. Getting a proper risk assessment cross-culturally is another problem. These are fundamental institutional building blocks that should be there. If 7% of inpatients would prefer to speak in another language, then you have to develop the capacity so they can have equitable care, which means you have to have an interpreting service that works."

Professor McKenzie's measured perspective seems to suggest that socio-economics and racism impact drastically on the mental health of African Caribbeans; that fear of mental health services inhibit African Caribbeans when it comes to engagement with these services; and that the inadaptable nature of the services offered, along with institutional racism, compound rather than cure mental illness among African Caribbean service users. So how best can these problems be addressed and solved? Not, according to Professor McKenzie, by *Delivering Race Equality,* but perhaps, ultimately, by hard-boiled economics. "The problem with DRE is people don't understand what it is. It's a policy document and a tool. For a tool and a policy document to have responsibility is part of the confusion. The responsibility rests squarely with the services under the Race Relations Amendment Act. DRE is an outline and a tool for people to actually keep their duties under the Race Relations Amendment Act. The fact that people don't do it is one of the reasons why the CRE is currently investigating the Department of Health. But they should be investigating mental health trusts. Trusts are given this money. They're supposed to provide equitable services under the Race Relations Amendments Act. They don't. There are stratagems in place that they could follow. And nobody does anything. That's the problem. I think the system is infinitely better than when I started psychiatry seventeen years ago. I think that DRE and things like that are things that only happen in the UK, because we do actually take it seriously. But I think that the CRE need to start thinking about how they're going to use the lever of the Race Relations Amendment Act to make public services do things. If the CRE decided to prosecute one trust, everybody else would do it. All it takes is the CRE to say, 'We're taking this seriously', then all of the other trusts would say, 'You know that document DRE? Why don't we actually bring it to life and do something? It's not like there's no information on how we should do it, it's not like we don't know the problems, but we actually need to get on and do this.' All public services have a race equality duty. They are supposed to seek out unlawful discrimination. They're supposed to offer equitable treatment. And they're supposed to promote racial equality as well. Each mental health trust is a public service and has a race equality duty. Most trusts don't actually fulfil their race equality duty. You're lucky if you've got a race equality scheme, let alone equitable services. Why would they, in the cash-strapped NHS, want to spend a lot of time producing equitable services? Unless somebody says, "We want you to show that you fulfil your race equality duty by producing proper services". If they decided to do that, then I think trusts would be more active and take it more seriously. If you think about it, if all the trusts were threatened with prosecution for not providing disability ramps, as soon as they thought that was going to happen, they'd think, right, ramps, when are we doing it? It can't be the responsibility of DRE to be the lever that makes people do their jobs. That's what the CRE and the Government are supposed to do. But with any group, across the whole BME population, I think that services will improve. The reason I think services will improve is that I think eventually it will dawn on the Government that it's cheaper to do it properly. By about 2030 or 2040, the majority of the working population in London will be from ethnic minorities. London's already about 30-35% ethnic minorities of working age. By that time it will be 52-53%. The powerhouse of the economy of the UK will be ethnic minority workers in London. Now you have a choice of people being ill and getting bad treatment, and therefore becoming economically inactive, or people getting ill and getting good treatment and staying economically active. The latter is the cheaper thing to do. And so I think we'll get into a position where, just like making sure all the young people didn't get TB so that we can send them out to war, which is what happened before World War II, we'll have a situation where people will say, "Actually, if we've got our workforce getting ill, and if we've got the problem of people staying in hospital at great expense, it's actually cheaper to go upstream and try and do some prevention work and produce better primary care and first contact services." In

Crisis in the Community

the long run a service like Antenna costs £300,000 a year. That's the same cost as two people ending up in a secure unit. In the end it is cheaper. Not only does that service prevent two people ending up in a secure unit, but if you then actually manage to get people early enough that they end up being economically active, then you save the exchequer a huge amount of money. The economic case for doing it properly is a no-brainer honestly. Humanity and social justice underlie a lot of the things people want to do. But in a complex society where there are loads of people vying for resources, and the press has a part to play in stigmatising particular groups, getting extra money for mental health services is always difficult. It isn't easy. And getting money for prevention and well being is also equally difficult. And getting money for ethnic minorities at the moment is difficult because of the discourse around failed asylum seekers. When you put it altogether, your ethnic minorities with mental health problems, and you're talking about prevention rather than anything else, it does become something that you're going to have to produce a number of arguments for to get the money that you need to do things. Of course it's an indictment of society. And of course everybody should have an ethical head on all the time, but they don't. And if the ethnical argument can't be joined, then you can say, 'Oh, and by the way, it costs you money'."

David Burke

Epilogue

At the time of this book's completion, the Government's new Mental Health Bill was fiercely criticised by professionals, race equality campaigners and human rights groups. Even the largely ineffectual Commission for Racial Equality and Human Rights joined the chorus of opposition; the bill, in its considered opinion, discriminated against ethnic minorities. A race equality impact assessment appended to the bill was, "At best flawed and at worst highly misleading". The commission went so far as to suggest the bill could be challenged by a judicial review.

Of particular concern was the extension of powers to detain and medicate individuals with supposedly dangerous views. It was feared such powers would be used to oppress people as a result of their political, religious and cultural beliefs. Matilda Macattram described community treatment orders as, "No more than psychiatric ASBOs, which have no place in mental health legislation", and which made, "Countless numbers of Black people prisoners in their own homes".

Marcel Vige, Chair of the National Black and Minority Ethnic Mental Health Network, claimed the bill would undermine Government efforts to improve mental health services through *Delivering Race Equailty*. And Professor Suman Fernando rejected an OBE in protest at the Government's

Crisis in the Community

failure to tackle racism in mental health services, charging that the bill had, "Dangerous implications for all of us, especially people from Black and Minority Ethnic communities". He said, "It seems most strange that the Government say they want to recognise my services to BME mental healthcare at a time when they are trying to push through legislation that would make things worse for Black people caught up in the mental health system, in spite of strong objections by many people, including myself, expressed both publicly and in private to Government ministers."

The struggle, it seems, is set to continue.